"*Survivors on the Yoga Mat* demonstrates beautifully how yoga can provide a pathway from pain and isolation to wholeness. Stories from a multiracial, intergenerational, cross-cultural group of people reveal the healing powers of yoga as widely accessible."—**Sharon Salzberg**, author of *Real Happiness at Work* and cofounder of the Insight Meditation Society

"This is the book I've been waiting for: a raw, real, and wonderful collection of stories to inspire all those who are on the pathway from trauma to transcendence."—**Nikki Myers**, yoga and somatic therapist and founder of Y12SR: The Yoga of 12-Step Recovery

"Most people assume that those of us that practice yoga are naturally calm and centered and have happened into equanimity in the same way that we might find a hundred dollar bill on the foot path. The truth is, many of us are drawn to yoga because of deep wounds and traumas that have not been resolved even after years of therapy. As Becky Thompson and her brave contributors relate, it is by entering into the world of body sensation, breath, and attention that we can move through and beyond the limited identity of a survivor into the truth of our boundless self. "—**Donna Farhi**, author of *Bringing Yoga to Life*

"A truly inspiring, informative, and important book! The process of meeting oneself at ever-deeper levels requires us to listen and follow our inner voice, taking courage to dive into our own personal journey through our practice. Becky Thompson shows us how to do this with sensitivity, clarity, and heart, demonstrating how asana, breath-work, and meditation are helping trauma survivors recover their power, their boundaries, and their joy in living fully and creatively."—**Angela Farmer**, world-renowned yoga teacher

"For survivors and those who love us: This book brings to light the patterns of entrapment that we all get tangled in. *Survivors on the Yoga Mat* documents that our pain, trauma, and wounds can be spoken, cleansed, sweat out, and released. *Survivors* brings deeper understanding to the journey through hell into power. May we all learn to Walk in Beauty."—**Ana Tiger Forrest**, author of *Fierce Medicine*

"Telling truthful stories is an essential act of activism … this book is full of them."—**Matthew Sanford**, president and CEO of Mind Body Solutions and author of *Waking*

"Yoga is for every body—young and old, Black as well as white. In this lovingly rendered book, Becky Thompson shows us that there are no limitations on who needs this ancient healing art and who can benefit from it."—**Jan Willis**, author of *Dreaming Me: Black, Baptist, and Buddhist—One Woman's Spiritual Journey.*

"It is rare to open a book and find stories that depict trauma as a great equalizer in the human experience. With the sterling voice of one who has been there, Becky Thompson has gifted us with fragrant balm for healing the soul. Whether or not we see ourselves as survivors of trauma, this book is a heartfelt guide to living awake in this body. At the end of a traditional Zen temple meal, we chant in gratitude, "May we exist in muddy water with purity like a lotus, thus we bow to Buddha." I bow to *Survivors on the Yoga Mat,* a garden of lotuses blossoming."—**Ryūmon Hilda Gutiérrez Baldoquín, Sensei;** editor of *Dharma, Color, and Culture: New Voices in Western Buddhism* and cofounder of Two Streams Zen

"*Survivors on the Yoga Mat* gives voice to those who, despite overwhelming odds, are choosing to return to Source moment by moment, breath by breath. These are stories of liberation in the deepest sense from extraordinary 'ordinary' folks who are using the ancient technology of yoga to transform their inner landscapes and step more fully and courageously into their lives."—**Keval Kaur Khalsa**, associate professor of the Practice of Dance & Theater Studies and director of the dance program at Duke University

"Everyone who has experienced tears and emotions on the mat will recognize themselves in this lovely book. Becky Thompson's tone is invitational; her language is soothing and clear; the wisdom she offers is affirming and validating. *Survivors on the Yoga Mat* will help students, teachers, and practitioners of all types of integrative therapies understand the the healing powers of a complete yoga practice."—**Kyczy Hawk**, author of *Yoga and the Twelve Step Path*

"In this genuine and personal account, Becky Thompson offers a variety of practical suggestions for using yoga as a companion to treatment for trauma."—**David Emerson**, author of *Overcoming Trauma through Yoga*

"I come from Sri Lanka, a land fondly remembered by its visitors as Paradise Island, but torn to pieces by thirty years of civil war and natural disasters such as tsunami. Reading Becky Thompson's *Survivors on the Yoga Mat* opens new horizons for my imagination, on how to live and work with the multiple survivors in my country, struggling to reach wholeness, but burdened with trauma. In *Survivors*, there is a thirst for holiness and wholeness, written by a human being with a heart for the universe, grounded on this 'common ground.'"
—**Sister Canice Fernando**, Sri Lanka

SURVIVORS
on the
Yoga Mat

Stories for Those Healing from Trauma

BECKY THOMPSON

Foreword by Rolf Gates

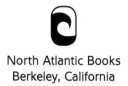

North Atlantic Books
Berkeley, California

Published by
North Atlantic Books
Huichin, unceded Ohlone land
aka Berkeley, California

Cover photo by Ernesto Galan
Cover and book design by Suzanne Albertson
Cover yogis: Becky Thompson and Wyoma

Photograph of Matcha Pornin on page 38 by Shelley Poplak. All other photos in the text and glossary by Ernesto Galan. All photography used with permission.

Printed in the United States of America

Survivors on the Yoga Mat: Stories for Those Healing from Trauma is sponsored and published by North Atlantic Books, an educational nonprofit based in the unceded Ohlone land Huichin (*aka* Berkeley, CA) that collaborates with partners to develop cross-cultural perspectives; nurture holistic views of art, science, the humanities, and healing; and seed personal and global transformation by publishing work on the relationship of body, spirit, and nature.

North Atlantic Books' publications are distributed to the US trade and internationally by Penguin Random House Publishers Services. For further information, visit our website at www.northatlanticbooks.com.

Library of Congress Cataloging-in-Publication Data
Thompson, Becky W.
    Survivors on the yoga mat: stories for those healing from trauma
    / Becky Thompson.
        pages cm
    Summary: "A collection of ninety true stories about how yoga can be used to work through past trauma; written by a trauma survivor and yoga instructor, designed as an inspirational guide for survivors practicing yoga as well as a resource for yoga teachers and therapists. Includes over 100 photos and descriptions of yoga postures mentioned in the book, as well as an appendix on the most popular schools of yoga and how their unique characteristics can be applied to psychological healing"— Provided by publisher.
    ISBN 978–1-58394–826–2 (paperback)
1. Post-traumatic stress disorder—Alternative treatment. 2. Yoga—Therapeutic use.
3. Psychotherapy. I. Title.
    RC552.P67T525 2014
    616.85'210642—dc23   2014006897

                    2 3 4 5 6 7 8 5LP 26 25 24 23 22

To Maury Stein, my first yogi
and Diane Harriford
"We shall call each other darling"

ACKNOWLEDGMENTS

I recently learned that a rainbow appears when sunlight bends as it enters a raindrop, touches the back of the drop, then bends again before it leaves, splitting its white light into red, orange, yellow, green, blue, and purple. This reminds me of yoga, how we enter the studio, touch the back of our own consciousness, and emerge changed. And it reminds me of writing this book—so many people doing back bends, forward bends, reverse warriors, and *tadasana* (ta-da!) to help make *Survivors* possible.

For beaming me support from the beginning, traveling together in this lifetime, I thank Diane Harriford. For so many conversations reflected in *Survivors* I thank the master gardener and poet Peg McAdam. Thank you to the various yoga studios—Bikram, Baptiste, Core Power, Down Under, the Daily Breath Yoga School, and the early dawn Forrest circle—for letting me be a yoga polygamist. Thank you to Samantha Cameron, Daniel Orlansky, Cat Kabira, and the team in Colorado Springs for your incredible teacher trainings. Thank you to Susan Kosoff, for Singapore in the summertime, we count this nine. To activist–scholar–life friend Monisha Das Gupta, namaste. Thank you to Sangeeta Tyagi; twenty-five years we call each other, "yes."

I give much appreciation to Joanne Wyckoff, whose humor, grace, and love of dancing makes working with an agent a truly lucky affair. Thank you to Mama Bear Betsy Rapoport, a creative coach with stellar ethics. Thanks to Beth Rathbaum, Brandi Perry, and Richard Tayson for your exquisite skills. And to all of the people at North Atlantic—including Jessica Sevey, Erin Wiegand, and Talia Shapiro—for your talented attention. Thanks to designer Suzanne Albertson, copyeditor Christopher Church, and indexer Ken DellaPenta for your generous work. Thank you to the Simmons librarians ("don't worry, we got this"), especially Dawn Stahura and Rex Krajewski. Thanks to the people at

Purple Cactus who laugh at my vegan requests ("seven blue corn chips"). Thank you to the Simmons College President's Fund for Faculty Excellence for travel and training. Namaste to many healer friends and colleagues: Cornell Coley, Desmond Patz, Wyoma, Nancy Shoemaker, Max Leeming, Valerie Leiter, Lisa Smith-McQueenie, Valerie Beaudrault, Zenaida Peterson, Ruthy Rickenbacker, Michele Berger, LaDonna Christian, Tricia Elam, and Karuna O'Donnell. Thank you to Ernesto "keep the edge" Galan for your talent and generosity as a photographer and to the illustrious crew of people whose poses bring such color and life to the book's glossary. We had way too much fun. Thanks to Abby Nathanson, publicity maven with so much flair.

Thank you to Maury Stein, Phyllis Stein, Morris Rabinowitz, and Cathy Colman for holding me. To Crystal, my daughter, who multiplies joy, for AcroYoga in swimming pools, bubble tea at the end of our days. To my son, LaMar, your heart so big. To my mother, sister, and brother, for blood that runs new. To Deborah, especially, for bringing celestial rhythms to our lucky days. Thank you to my grandmother, her spirit, my backbone, her last journey, a practice in love. To the ancestors and spirits, "[bearing] witness // within us // to all that we are // aware."[1]

I am grateful to the people in the United States, Thailand, Singapore, Bali, Cuba, Egypt, and Costa Rica who have shared their yoga and healing stories; your resilience and vulnerability, double gifts. And to the luminous crew at the Dorchester YMCA each week, hero's pose is an asana in your name. Thank you as well to so many yogi authors, in particular the big thinker Amy Weintraub and to Rolf Gates, whose *Meditations from the Mat* has been a marvelous model. I am also grateful to Ouyporn Khuankaew and Ginger Norwood, founders of the International Women's Partnership for Peace and Justice in Thailand. Their community-based retreat center is a precious gift for the world; teaching with them, a practice in bliss.

For you, dear reader, whom I have been writing to in my dreams, on trips, in the bathtub, and at the desk, please read as you want, in whatever order you desire. Part prayer, part story, part question, part plea, these entries were written for you. May they be sweet company for you as you have been for me. Thank you for being out there, willing to read.

CONTENTS

PART III

Hide and Seek: The Circuitous Path of Healing 77

PART IV

The Color of Rothko's Blue: Long-Term Wholeness 113

PART V

In the Shadow of the Temple: The Special Work of Teachers 147

PART VI

"Love Calls Us to the Things of This World": Yoga and Activism 180

FOREWORD

I can see Monterey Bay from my house, the expanse of ocean and the mountains surrounding it. I gaze out on it every day that I can, and I often think about the surf innovator Jack O'Neill, who looked out on this same unexplored wilderness and dreamed of an adventure we could all go on. Sixty years later countless people have been able to explore the ocean outside their door because Jack O'Neill explored the ocean outside his. I feel as though Becky Thompson is like Jack O'Neill. She has explored the ocean of her own heart, and I believe countless people will be aided in exploring theirs by reading this book. Becky Thompson has put two words together that represent a new possibility in human potential, *yoga* and *survivor*.

When I hear the word *survivor* I think of the ways I have made my life worth living when it felt like it wasn't. I think of the ways I have found hope when there was none, joy when there was none, love when there was none. I think of the worlds I created for myself when it felt like there was no place for me in this one. I think of a child's imagination, a child's heart, a child's tenderness, a child's playfulness, a child's ability to forgive. I think of our ability to endure. I think of what it means to be resilient.

There is a special beauty that a survivor creates; she is an artist whose canvas is her living, and the colors she uses are her smile, her joy, her laughter, her ease, her generosity, her courage, her kindness, her honesty, her ability to love wholeheartedly. This is the only beauty I have ever known. My parents are survivors, and so am I. I have traveled almost exclusively in the worlds survivors have made for themselves. When I needed to learn how to use drugs to live another day, survivors taught me how to get high. When I needed to learn how to get off drugs to live another day, survivors taught me how to get sober. When it was not enough to have survived, survivors taught me how to live. When I lost loved ones, survivors taught me how to grieve. When my wife and I chose not to raise our children as survivors, survivors taught me how to love. When I looked for something to do with my life, saying thank you to the countless survivors who have helped me along the way gave me a purpose.

Being a survivor is not a box I live in, however; it is a step I stand on as I live into a life second to none. Survivors taught me this. We are not without choice; we do not have to live in the shadow world of our pasts, acting out the same dramas again and again; we can choose to let go of the past, live into the light, and find our home there.

This is what it means to understand yoga, finding one's home in this breath, this body, this moment. When I hear the word *yoga* I see sunlight coming through the window of a sacred space. I hear fall leaves moving to a gentle breeze under a blue sky. I feel a summer lake tickling my ankles, its surface a miraculous glassy reflection of the mountains around it. I remember a room full of people taking the first deep breath they'd had all day. I experience a joy too big to name that is spreading from one heart to the next. I know the eternal moment is my home and I want nothing more.

My experience of surviving is that it is what I did to stay alive until I learned to love and to be loved. Yoga has been essential to this learning process, and I know that Becky Thompson's work will help yours. She has combined all of the essential ingredients. In this book you will find kindness, honesty, humility, clarity, experience, facts, poetry, humor, and the power of many voices raised to raise the human spirit. It is an honor to have been able to be a part of this great work. May you be safe, may you be healthy, may you be happy, may you know freedom, find peace, and walk through the world with ease.

Awake in truth together,
Rolf Gates, author of *Meditations from the Mat*

INTRODUCTION

In the last twenty years there has been a dramatic rise in our understanding of trauma. At the same time, the number of yoga studios popping up all over the country makes yoga look like the new Starbucks on the block. These two trends have converged in interesting ways, with research from the last decade revealing what many yoga practitioners have long known: yoga heals. Recent studies involving veterans, refugees, incest survivors, people paralyzed in accidents, and many other trauma survivors are confirming the power of yoga as a tool of healing not just for physical problems but for psychological and emotional injuries. Leading yoga retreat centers—Kripalu Center, the Omega Institute, and others—are beginning to recognize the need for trauma-sensitive training, a reality that will eventually enable a new generation of teachers to be well versed in the complexities of working with trauma survivors.

One early inspiration for writing *Survivors on the Yoga Mat* came while I was participating in a yoga teacher training. During the training I realized that we attendees were paying almost no attention to yoga's possible effects on trauma survivors. And yet, in the course of the training, I watched some of the participants struggle—dissociating during sessions;[1] whispering in the halls afterward about flashbacks, memories, and scary feelings; bingeing to numb those feelings; struggling with depression. I myself had been thrown back into feelings of being trapped and smothered during a session when we were practicing Thai massage on each other—all feelings I had faced during sexual abuse as a child. But no one, it seemed, felt comfortable talking publicly about these issues.

Caught off guard by the vulnerability I felt during that training, I co-led a workshop on trauma, knowing that, if we, as seasoned practitioners, were having trouble speaking openly about the process of healing from trauma, it must be all the more terrifying for people new to yoga. For the workshop, my collaborator and I brought in cutting-edge medical research that revealed yoga's healing powers, and this material opened people's minds. But what I found myself craving that day was an accessibly written, intimate book of stories about trauma survivors that I could share with people to illuminate the often circuitous and ingenious ways by which people use yoga in their journey toward healing.[2]

This is what birthed this book. *Survivors on the Yoga Mat* consists of one- to three-page stories, vignettes, and musings—alternately irreverent, funny, serious, insightful, and surprising. These brief reflections, which are organized into six sections, can be read sequentially or as freestanding entries. If you are like me, you will skip around the book, letting your interests guide you. But you can read the entries in order, too, following the chronological sequence of the book from early yoga practice to yoga as a lifetime journey. You can read the reflections while on a city bus or subway, when you are having a bad hair day, when you are lonely, late at night, or when you want to feel like you are still in the realm of yoga when you are not on the mat. Or, you can keep the book close by but just peek in when you can. That's okay, too.[3] The format of the book speaks to a twenty-first-century audience, a culture on the go more likely to read a blog than a novel, to those who gather knowledge on the run.

About one-quarter of the entries draw on my own story as a trauma survivor. While much of my writing over the years has focused on trauma, I have rarely put my own story on the page. I have to admit, doing so hasn't been easy. In fact, an editor of an earlier version of *Survivors* kindly noted that I was tucking my own story behind the others even as I thought I was already taking up too much space on the page. For me, the stacking of traumas before I was five years old left me with a wobbly sense of myself. Born into a Mormon family in Utah and raised in Arizona, I was brought into the world by two teen parents who had more than their share of demons dogging them. Early trauma included being sexually abused, which left me with a torn-up sense of my own bodily parameters. I was exposed to parental alcoholism, physical abuse, and witnessing my father, whom I adored, try to kill himself. Trauma in adolescence included molestation by my mother's live-in boyfriend, another divorce, and increasing clues that I was not okay (starving myself, bingeing, believing I needed to perform sexually, and being afraid to trust anyone).

In early adulthood I found a therapist who knew to diagnose me with post–traumatic stress disorder (PTSD) before that diagnosis was commonly used. Her naming was a relief, helping me confess to her why my wanting to exit the world might make sense. We worked on the later years—the second incest, the parental alcoholism, a second divorce—before I could touch what happened before I was in kindergarten.

Once I found yoga, the practice helped me heal in ways talk therapy could not, since memories were stuck in my body in places no words alone could find. Some of what I have recovered still feels incoherent, like I am making it up. My continued love for my mother makes naming these traumas in print hard—I honestly know she did her best given her own traumatized history. But this is no distanced, academic book. I write as someone who was outside of my body (and away from my feelings) for much of my life, who still struggles with "fat" brain (thinking I am the size of a puffy monster), who routinely blames myself, who sometimes walks toward unsafe people rather than away from them, who still pushes too hard. All along, I have been less interested in blaming people for past injuries and more keen on feeling whole. But I can't write about trauma and its consequences as something "over there." For years, looking up at the yoga studio ceiling during practice made me feel sick, the texture of its bumpy surface reminding me of the Styrofoam-turned-to-cement feel of my body after sexual abuse. For years in yoga I thought of any excuse imaginable to leave before the final resting posture, the idea of lying still (with rage, sadness, loneliness bumping around in my body) easily sending me into a panic. For me, and many others, dissociation is the norm, not the exception, splitting into multiple parts a way we protect ourselves against dissolving completely.

While I worry that sharing my story might contribute to a society obsessed with confession, another part of me knows that it is in the details that we often come to recognize each other and ourselves. As the singer Holly Near once said, "linger on the details, the part that reflects the change."[4] When it comes to trauma, the first and last thing we need to do is make room for specificity. It is the specific memories, images, and nightmares that need to find air.

In *Survivors* I write about the quiet focus that yoga nurtures and that I can now take into my teaching and writing; about the voluminous life force energy *(prana)* stirred up by yoga that I experience in my teaching and activism; about the alternately moving and hilarious lessons that I learn from students in my classes; and most of all about how yoga helps trauma survivors find the strength to "carry the sky on our heads" (in the words of a creation myth from the people of Guinea).[5]

While it took me years of practicing yoga before I began to understand why teachers always stress breathing, I now know how conscious breathing can keep me from flying apart when things are difficult, can anchor me to moments of peace. Yoga helped me through the days and months after my adopted son left when he was thirteen to live with his biological mom, the light on his Game Boy still lit in my mind. The steadiness of mind that comes with long-term practice keeps me calm even when a wound-up world threatens to hot press my days. Over the years, yoga has also brought me joy and a connection to an ever-expanding network of people who stretch their way past tired and hurt into places of energy and insight.

While I weave autobiographical details throughout the book, the bulk of the entries are sparked by stories from students I have worked with, friends, writers, activists, and people I have met on my travels: a high school heroin addict who is now a revered yoga teacher; a poet and a vet whose writing teaches us about heartbreak and healing; a Buddhist on death row whose time on the cushion spurs him to interrupt the murder of a gay inmate; a firefighter who moonlights as a generous and fun-loving yoga instructor; a professor who links her agitation during sitting meditation to the ceaseless movement of her people during the Great Migration.[6] The complicated, often wry insights of these practitioners counter the all-too-precious elitism that many associate with yoga practice. And their stories also reveal great patience—the patience to come to the mat even when everything is churning inside; the patience to view scary memories as tender friends; and ultimately the patience to know and accept that some things can never be made right.

The people whose stories are recounted in the book explain why "living in the body"[7] takes guts, why survivors are close cousins to cats with nine lives, why healing can make living through a hurricane seem easy. These people include some who have a practice made up of poses *(asanas)* as well as those whose practice involves other aspects of the eight-limbed spiritual path first outlined by philosopher Patanjali in the third century BCE. (See appendix I for a diagram of these limbs in English and Sanskrit, appendix II for a glossary of the poses).[8] These limbs include the laws of life *(yamas)*, the rules for living *(niyamas)*, the postures *(asanas)*, mindful breathing *(pranayama)* turning inward *(pratyahara)*, concentration *(dharana)*, meditation *(dhyana)*, and the cultivation of bliss *(samadhi)*.[9] In this book, attention is on yoga in the big sense of the word—not only the practice of specific physical postures but also on other yogic practices that enable inner growth and spiritual awakening.

The stories told in the book include those by people who have lived through war; sexual, physical, and emotional abuse; loss of a loved one; mental or physical illness; racism, poverty, and homophobia; incarceration; and human-made and natural disasters. While the diversity of experience among survivors makes generalizations about us difficult, we do seem to have some shared characteristics worth noting. Most survivors have found it difficult to live comfortably in our own bodies. This may date back to episodes of sexual abuse when the mind left the body behind in order to get through the horror of what was taking place, or to terrifying flashbacks related to combat, accidents, or natural disasters. Whatever the source of the disconnection from the body, many of us come to yoga seeking ways to experience our bodies as safe and welcoming again.

People who are healing from trauma also tend to struggle with being able to say what we feel, a problem that yoga can help to heal over time. One of the common characteristics of trauma is its overwhelming nature—the events are so over-the-top in terms of danger and pain that it is hard at the time to stay with one's feelings, to "process" the event. Anyone who has ever done an extended backbend or stayed in a difficult pose for a long time knows yoga's power to make us feel again, even as these feelings can be overwhelming.

Survivors on the Yoga Mat was written for those of us with the wiggles—those who dread the meditation at the end—"What, you want me to sit still?"—as well as those who count the minutes until they can finally lie down and rest. It is for people who have a hard time finding the motivation to even get to the mat, for those who cry between poses, who hide our faces as tears stream down during the final meditation, for those who have been unable to cry for years, and also for those who haven't yet arrived at the mat. This book is for those who are self-conscious about moving, about showing up in class not knowing how to hold our bodies, who try to be as invisible as possible, slipping in and out of class without anyone noticing. It is for those who have been brave enough to try to stay present during practice, even when difficult feelings arise. It is for those who tried yoga and then had to back off for a while, when symptoms of chronic fatigue or lupus make coming to the mat too physically risky. And it is for anybody who loves survivors, who walks beside us and has faith in our ability to heal. If there is one message that I hope this book conveys, it is that healing takes place within communities of people who support us.

Though I reference some of the current scientific research on yoga, trauma, and healing, *Survivors on the Yoga Mat* isn't an exhaustive study. Nor do I wish to present myself as yoga's cheerleader, for I know that there is no single way that people heal from trauma and that some of yoga's current orthodoxies don't work so well for certain survivors. Rather, I think of the book as a series of reflections by a woman who is a trauma survivor as well as a scholar, poet, mother, and teacher who wants yoga to be available to people who would find it helpful, but who also knows that survivors are a special bunch in terms of how we see the world. This is sometimes a blessing and sometimes a curse. We can be acutely sensitive, and easily hurt; we can be exquisitely alert but also seek ways to numb out; we are remarkably empathetic, but we sometimes expect the world to read our minds.

I wrote *Survivors on the Yoga Mat* for people who practice yoga, mindfulness, and meditation, but a background in those areas is by no means essential. While the book is steeped in my awareness of current research, you don't need to be a trauma survivor, or even someone with a particular interest in trauma, to appreciate it. As I was writing the book, I deliberately asked careful readers who are neither yoga practitioners nor trauma survivors to give me their opinions to be sure that anyone who picks up the book will see a part of themselves in the stories.

The stories include everyday people squeezing yoga practice between work and picking up Popeye's chicken for the kids on the way home. My main goals are to bring to life the courage and persistence of those who have used yoga to heal themselves, and through them to inspire others to investigate yoga's healing powers. In that way, the book was written for survivors as well as health professionals (doctors, therapists, body workers, and physical therapists), trauma researchers, and educators. I hope it speaks to yoga teachers; those interested in spirituality and meditation; dancers, athletes, and other body-practitioners who seek to know the body's pleasures and beauty; poets, writers, and readers of spirituality and health-related memoirs; and social activists seeking ways to sustain our work mindfully.

In my years as a teacher and practitioner, what I have loved is how spacious yoga can be. With the students I have encountered both in Boston and in the places my travels have taken me, I have found that the poses offer a language that goes deeper than words, a way of living that speaks to people across many cultures and borders. The main principles of yoga (nonviolence, self-reflection, valuing simplicity and contentment, honesty, integrity), which are universal, have been guides that I keep close to my heart and try to practice in my life—whether teaching college, talking with my daughter, mourning a loss, or just being stalled in traffic. Over the years, I have gone to the mat many times feeling like I could cry. Sometimes I still feel like that even after practice. Mostly, though, I have seen a deepening and widening of what feels like safety in my life, a healing I try to convey in the entries that follow.

It is this commitment to healing that we take with us when looking for the right yoga teachers and traditions. Given the growing range of yoga approaches available to us, it can take effort and patience to find the right

match (see appendix III). The right fit has to do with whether the fundamental approach works for you. (Is it lively or quiet, vigorous or relaxing,
practiced in a hot room or a cooler space, athletic or spiritual, involving
detailed instruction or more self-initiative?) The teacher's personality,
experience, and approach—how you feel as you are learning—also makes
a big difference. While it may help if the teacher has had some experience
working with trauma survivors, and it is certainly your right to ask about
that, basic kindness, attentiveness, sensitivity, intuition, and creativity can
go a long way to helping survivors heal ourselves.

For sure, it is acceptable to speak up or leave a class if something
upsets you. Of course you have the right (and it is gutsy) to be upfront
with a teacher about your struggles or worries. You also have the right
to say nothing at all, to feel your way through practices until you want
to talk. With yoga, we get to decide when to stay and when to go. Where
you end up—a gentle class with soothing music or a highly structured
practice with a fired-up instructor—can be surprising. Who knew *that*
would work? And what might be right for several years can change over
time. So, as is true for many things, flexibility and a beginner's mind
remain essential. But if survivors are anything, we are willing, creative,
and resilient to the bone.

This book's six parts travel from early yoga challenges and discover-
ies to musings about how the practice of yoga can heal us both on and
off the mat. Each section opens with an introduction that provides the
framework for the entries that follow. Part I, "Deeper than Words," offers
a number of stories describing what brings those who have been traumatized to the mat. Part II, "Like Dragonflies," focuses on what makes trauma
survivors distinctive, how our abilities and challenges shape the way we
practice yoga, the way we are in the world. The title of this section is from
the poet Martín Espada, drawing a parallel between trauma survivors
and dragonflies—with their multifaceted large eyes and iridescent wings
that are always outstretched. The title of part III, "Hide and Seek," alludes
to how healing from trauma is often touch and go, not logical or easily
measured. Sometimes healing presents itself like a flock of landing geese.
Sometimes it is as elusive as a single hummingbird at night.

Part IV, "The Color of Rothko's Blue," takes its title from the gorgeous color in Mark Rothko's paintings, which I see as the expanded consciousness that emerges when one practices yoga consistently. The long-term benefits from yoga come not only from stretching and breathing but also from committing oneself to self-reflection. The stories in this section speak to the discipline that healing requires, how the practice of yoga widens and deepens over time. Part V, "In the Shadow of the Temple," illuminates the special work of teachers—the confident, tender, listening, fierce, marvelous, gutsy, innovative qualities that they bring to their work with survivors. The stories illustrate what survivors can learn from teachers and teachers from survivors, and what happens when a person is both. The final section, which takes its title from a Richard Wilbur poem, "Love Calls Us to the Things of This World," speaks to the potential for yoga to be both a space of personal revelation and a way of transforming the world.

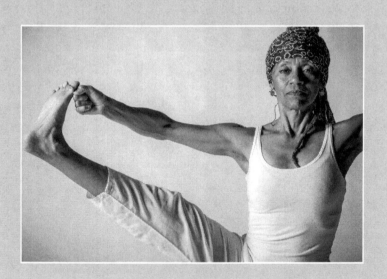

PART I

Deeper than Words

Finding the Mat

Many trauma survivors come to our first yoga class not quite knowing what brought us here. Perhaps a friend dragged us, or we stumbled across a coupon that meant trying yoga was simply too cheap to pass up. Or maybe we noticed something different in our friend who had been doing yoga for a while, some inexplicable ease when he laughed, a certain lightness in his gait when he crossed the room. But we don't really know why we have come and once here, we may feel even less clear about why we are staying. Who needs it?

When I first started coming to yoga classes in my late thirties, I wasn't sure why either. I did know that after working with two gifted therapists, much of the healing I still needed to do couldn't be done with words. The trauma—particularly the sexual abuse and exposure to violence I faced when very young—needed to move around in my body and then be released. At the time, however, the notion of "finding it in my body" felt so vague to me that stepping out of the realm of talk therapy and into that of movement sounded more like a crazy leap of faith than anything else.

Nonetheless, I took that leap. At forty, I decided I was going to pretend that I was thirty-five so I could live the past five years over again. In my mind, five seemed about the right number of years to represent the toll that trauma had exacted. Magical thinking, I know, to believe I could assign a number to the cost of trauma, but I decided that for each found year—thirty-five to forty—I would add a new body-based practice to my yoga practice, starting the first year with working with a personal trainer, then adding salsa, then merengue and bachata, then, as it turns out, more yoga. Lots more yoga.

Looking back on what I did, I can see how each body practice was helping me build toward wholeness. At the time, though, I couldn't yet see the pattern. In finding a personal trainer to work with me at the gym, I had someone who, three times a week, would focus on me, only me, watch and coach and witness and laugh and encourage me as my lower back got stronger (i.e., I became better able to stand up for myself), my arm muscles developed (which means I gained the confidence to wear sleeveless shirts), and my abs got stronger (which helped keep my back pain-free during long hours at my desk). And I loved the music playing at the gym—Aretha Franklin, Beyoncé, Chaka Khan, Luther, Santana, Nellie—jamming, filling me up with rhythm and melody, all before 8 o'clock in the morning.

After a year of gym training, I started taking salsa lessons, no small thing since my relatives and I refer to Mormonism as the "ironing board" culture—hold your body as erect as possible and don't breathe. No movement, no joy, and certainly no dance. Salsa didn't come easily to me, unlike many of the twenty-something women in the class who appeared to have been dancing since birth. They would twirl themselves around, doing triple turns and back bends that looked like magic to me, as I painstakingly practiced my once-around, find-a-point-without-getting-dizzy steps. It helped to have a compassionate Guatemalan dance instructor who would sometimes whirl me around the dance floor, making me temporarily look better than I was. And, over time, especially when I danced with someone I could relax with, I started to improve.

My first exposure to yoga was a Bikram class that became a steady practice for seven years. Then I branched out—to Vinyasa Flow, Forrest Yoga, Iyengar-based practice, Kundalini, and Shakti yoga dance.[1] Along the way, I began to teach as well, as I started to see a connection between moving my body and memory, between practicing postures and feeling, between postures and finding ways to be in the world where I wasn't always afraid. Gradually yoga became a practice toward which the whole of my being gravitated. Over time, my study of yoga philosophy increased too, as did my understanding of the links between the physical postures and the other limbs of yoga. I sought out people who were practicing the eight limbs of yoga, especially those who were unabashedly seeking bliss *(samadhi)*.

My journey has been a feeling one, during which I have been, at different times, both as vulnerable and as resilient as a winter rose. An early, emblematic yoga memory: doing camel pose *(ustrasana),* that intense, heart-opening backbend, and coming up from it sobbing, only to hear the teacher, Diane Ducharme, say that, "feelings come up in camel that you might not expect. They are normal. Crying on the mat is okay." The first time I heard these words, I thought she was saying them just for me—that she saw my tears and was trying to comfort me. It took me a while to understand that her words reflect the compassion of many yoga instructors and that the reaction I was having, others have had, too. The floor series, especially the postures involving various kinds of backbends—physical postures that tapped into my fears of being alone and unsafe that I thought I had dealt with but clearly had not—made me see that memories were lurking in my body. For survivors of traumas that had taken place prior to our ability to talk, healing means getting in touch with what the body knew before words. I was starting to realize that healing meant finding in the body the self that existed before trauma, the self that changed during the trauma, and the self that had come out the other side dazed, and often driven. Such healing also required that I start reaching out, that I look into the glistening eyes of others who were struggling both on and off the mat but still, sometimes miraculously, coming back to it.

The stories in this section give glimpses of early doubts about yoga, early realizations, and early joys. Being able to stay on the mat and develop a consistent practice means moving through postures—particularly the aptly named heart-opening asanas—that may bring up far more emotions than we bargained for. Meditation can be challenging for similar reasons, on top of which it involves sitting still, which for some of us is almost impossible. Even the injunction of the yoga teacher to breathe consciously, in and out, can be terrifying, as revealed in the story about a woman whose childhood bouts of asthma often left her gasping for breath, petrified that she would not be able to get enough oxygen to survive.

Many people come to yoga with a sense that something important is missing in their lives, only to discover that the work of finding what they lost is arduous, the physical postures in yoga only one small piece of the work to be done. In early yoga the predictability and dedication of longtime yogis may not at first appeal to the restless and reckless among us, but gradually the discipline involved begins to make more sense. Early yoga reminds us that we are all beginners, practicing with a body that changes every day, and with a mind that may be changing every day, too. As weeks of yoga turn into months and then years, yoga practitioners begin to see life changing, the consistency of practice bringing new kindness to people's days.

"The Door Itself Makes No Promises"

Either you will
go through this door
or you will not go through.

If you go through
there is always the risk
of remembering your name.

Things look at you doubly
and you must let them look back
and let them happen.

If you do not go through
it is possible
to live worthily

to maintain your attitudes
to hold your position
to die bravely

but much will blind you,
much will evade you,
at what cost who knows?

The door itself
makes no promises.
It is only a door.
　　　—Adrienne Rich[2]

Going through the door to a yoga class for the first time is no small endeavor. You may worry about what to wear and whether everyone else will be able to pretzel themselves into poses as you stand there rigid as a stick. You may be anxious about going into a room where you will be the only person who isn't white, or young, or female, or spandex-clad, or thin and lithe as a ballet dancer. Maybe the teacher will correct your posture in front of the class, or maybe you will pass out from the heat.

Or perhaps you are simply concerned that you will be wasting your time, since counting calories burned at the gym has been the primary way you measure the value of any physical activity. Or you might wonder if doing yoga will take you away from your responsibilities—your children, your work, your activist commitments.

Beyond these concerns there may lie deeper ones. You may sense that sitting quietly in meditation, lying in corpse pose *(savasana),* or moving through the poses will bring up emotions long buried. A lot of people know—whether consciously or not—that they have for years, sometimes decades, staggered under troubles that are too heavy to be carried, too frightening to be spoken of, too coded, too layered, too buried to be allowed to emerge. So you lug around these troubles, a weight that never appears on the scales but only in the workings of your heart, your soul, your body. You can still live your life carrying your troubles, "but," as Adrienne Rich writes, "much will blind you, // much will evade you, // at what cost who knows? // The door itself // makes no promises. // It is only a door."

That is the truth about yoga, too. It makes no immediate promises. Why, then, is it worth driving to the studio after work instead of going to a bar? What is the point of spending one long weekend at a meditation retreat instead of staying home with loved ones? What is the value of teenagers attending a community-run yoga class? Will doing yoga help stop the violence in their neighborhoods, prevent their friends from getting shot?

You might also wonder, "Is it worth it to simply close my eyes, get still, and do 'nothing' while the rest of my life is running away with itself?"

Yoga gives you a portal to knowledge that you have stored in your bodies but have not known how to access. It gives you ways to handle difficulties that may be clouding your eyes and silencing your tongue, creates a certain distilled awareness that allows you to unscramble your brain, and when the time is right, let go of the burden you have carried so long.

The therapist I worked with throughout my twenties, a woman who had also faced serious challenges growing up, had a mantra that she passed on to me: "I will remember everything I know and know everything I remember." Yoga helps with that deep recall. Helps you face your fears, unseal your lips, get and stay active in your communities, become proactive in the name of peace.

The Body Remembers

Many yoga masters, yoga therapists, and somatic psychologists
believe that everything we've ever experienced is stored in the body.
Even when traumatic memory is repressed, the body remembers.
—Amy Weintraub[3]

Years ago, when I was on a book tour traveling from city to city, I found
myself trying to explain to people who had not experienced trauma what
it is like for those who have.[4] Describing common responses to trauma—
dissociation, numbness, isolation—seemed to get me part way there, but
I was having a difficult time helping people *feel* what it is like. Eventually,
I started to explain the aftermath of trauma this way: imagine that you
are driving to your house. You turn onto the street where you live and are
just about to pull into your driveway when you realize that your house is
not there any more. It is missing, a big space where your house used to
be. You get out of the car, in shock and panic, wondering what to do. It
occurs to you that someone in the neighborhood might have seen what
happened to your house, who took it, where it went, so you go door-to-
door, asking, "Remember my house? It's gone. Do you remember seeing
it? Do you know what happened to it? Is there anyone else who might
have seen it?" If nobody gives you a satisfactory answer, it might occur
to you to call the police, report a missing house, hoping that they have a
division for such things and are willing to send someone out to witness
the hole where your house used to be.

This is what it is like for many people who have been traumatized.
We run around trying to find a witness. We try to find people who
remember the house before it went missing, who will know who we
were before the trauma. If we find someone who saw the house before it
was stolen, we might grill them with questions, somehow thinking that
if we can discover the facts of the story, we will begin to understand.
If we do find an eyewitness, we might also be able to talk about what
we miss about the house and our possible next steps. If we can't find
a witness, though, that void can feel disorienting. It can start to make

us wonder if we invented the house, if we simply made up the story we have been telling ourselves.

For people who have been traumatized through child abuse, incest, war, political torture, or police brutality, it might never be possible to find a reliable witness, someone who was there who can tell you what happened, who can identify the perpetrator. This reality is one of the many reasons that getting to the mat helps. You may never know who hurt you, why they hurt you, or even exactly how they hurt you. You may never be able to remember the actual moments when the house was stolen, when the physical structure that housed your spirit was moved, taken, went missing. But there is something about getting into child's pose *(balasana)* day after day, hoisting ourselves up into headstands *(sirsasana)*, finding an alignment in pigeon *(eka pada raja kapotasana)* that helps build a new house—one that no one can ever take away since it is inside of us, built molecule by molecule from the inside out.

In yoga practice we find witnesses, teachers, and fellow mat lovers who see us rebuilding, watch us crow *(bakasana)*, and toe stand *(padangustasana)* our way through to memory, to awareness, to wholeness.

We Were Taught to Forget

> The practice of Yoga helps us connect with the part of ourselves that is always virgin and untouched: the place within us that can never be damaged.
> —Donna Farhi[5]

When I was a child, I was sure I could fly. I flew in my dreams and thought I could when I was awake, too, but I somehow knew not to tell people, thinking that they might not believe me. Not surprisingly, at some point along the way of traumas coming my direction, I stopped flying and even forgot that I could until, in my mid-twenties, I joined a women's spirituality group. Looking back, this is when yoga began for me, way before I was introduced to the postures.

In this group, the high priestess would lead us on these guided visualizations where we were asked to go to a safe place as she talked us through the ritual. Most of the time I fell fast asleep during these meditations, waking only when the leader started beckoning us back into the room. I remember worrying that people would make fun of me for missing out on the whole experience. I didn't know how to say that closing my eyes and letting my mind wander or settle was entirely too threatening to me, entirely unsafe. Tellingly, the times that I did stay awake, when the leader asked us to visualize a safe space, most of the women in the group went to quiet places in nature—the dunes in Provincetown, the Grand Canyon, a forest in Vermont. Meanwhile, I imagined myself in Downtown Crossing in Boston, one of the busiest urban spaces in the city, teeming with street venders selling sausage and popcorn, businesspeople grabbing lunch between meetings, pigeons claiming their pecking space on the cobblestones, teenagers running around enjoying a day of skipping school.

In the visualization, I sat right on a bench, absorbing the smells, rhythms, street music, that space a safe one for me since there were so many people there who could be my witness, who reminded me I was alive. I remember feeling defensive about my visualized space of choice, thinking that it revealed my jumbled, skittery consciousness. I was not defensive, however, when, about a year into our meetings, I was able to announce that I had begun flying again in my dreams. I was beginning to find powers of perception buried somewhere between daddy one and daddy two, between incest and drinking, between clenching and dread, as my mother worked to keep herself and her children afloat. I was beginning to know where I was coming from, where I had been.

Trauma may not only make people afraid to look backward (afraid of what we might remember and feel again). It can also make looking forward seem scary (worried that we might not have the skills, the companionship, the growth we will need in the future). This dual reality ironically keeps us perched in a limbo state disconnected from the past or future. Part of the beauty of yoga, whether it be through meditation or postures, is its ability to help us bypass the tricks that our minds play on us, to get to the expanded consciousness that lived within us before damage was done. The joy of that journey is its ability to be more integrated in the present, to bring to consciousness the beauty we always knew about ourselves but were taught to forget. This is what yoga promises as we begin to stretch between forward and backward bends, seeking a place right in between, in the present, the beauty of that space.

Renegade Memory

The growing movement among neuroscientists to understand how healing is occurring in the brain through extensive yoga and meditation is showing that a healthy, balanced use of the brain is one where the left and right brain are connected, where one does not override or trump the other. For trauma survivors, such a state of balance is a challenge. Healing requires us to move implicit memory (renegade, flashback memory) that is housed in the right brain to explicit memory in the left brain in order to then develop narrative integration (stories that make some sense, that bring a sense of order and understanding).[6] The left and right brain have to link in order to create a coherent narrative. When a memory is not yet integrated, it is stored in the right brain and is largely unconscious. The right brain sends what is essentially gobbledygook to the left hemisphere. This is nonintegrated memory. Resolution of trauma occurs when the left and right brain are working together with the emotions attached.

Yoga can heal partly because it requires a balanced use of the left and right brain. While practicing, we are processing language, making analytical links between postures, and aware of our own narrator that is witnessing and chronicling the practice. At the same time, the right brain is rapidly firing—tapping into body memory, the unconscious, the land of sensation, and deep awareness. This allows us to be in our bodies as we practice. That is what is sometimes called being in the flow—that delicious time of integration and balance.

I witnessed a powerful example of how yoga can help with memory retrieval and brain integration through a story told to me by Jazz, a lesbian activist and yoga practitioner I met in Thailand. For the longest time during practice, Jazz felt afraid if anyone came close to touching her stomach. Oftentimes she would also need to sit up during practice for fear of how she might feel when lying down with her stomach exposed. She didn't know why she had these symptoms or what they meant. Then, when her niece confided that her father, Jazz's brother, had been raping her, Jazz realized for the first time that he had raped her, too. She began to understand that the pain she felt if a teacher touched her abdomen or a posture required her stomach to be exposed related to unconscious memories that had been stored in her stomach all those years. It took her niece's story and Jazz's outrage to get in touch with the rape memory archived in her body. In that moment, the renegade memory began to be integrated into her consciousness—a left and right brain link that allowed her to take further steps in healing. With this awareness she began confiding in her lover about the link between the pain in her stomach and its traumatic roots. And she began to see yoga as a healing practice since the sensations she had in her body could give her clues to what she had experienced and repressed.

For many people, healing from trauma involves a consistent practice where we can experience this flow—this right- and left-brain integration. In my own case, this integration has facilitated a more coherent narrative about my life. The panic I have experienced in a hot yoga room, especially if I was not by the door or a window, felt a lot like being locked in a basement where there was not enough air or light (which a relative did to my sister and me when we were very young). The fear I felt when a teacher would make an assist from behind without notice was reminiscent of being hit from behind by a parent when I was a child. Identifying my reactions to a hot room or an unannounced assist helped me turn renegade memories (flashbacks) into explicit memory. And, perhaps more importantly, I began to see that I have survived feelings of being trapped or caught off guard. My feelings come from somewhere—they belong to experiences I lived through before—but they do not have to rule me now.

Left and right brain integration has given me a better ability to steady myself when something catches me off guard. I can watch the emotions and then try to understand why I may be reacting that way. My thinking feels more balanced and my posture is better (after years of standing at a kind of tilt, a little perched to the left). I now understand that twenty-plus years of migraines partly related to living in my head, not in my body. Part of the beauty of yoga is how much it requires me to develop right brain capacities since earlier in my life I mostly lived in the land of the left brain (highly analytical, logical, and categorical). Spending much of the last fifteen years hanging out with the right side of my brain has helped balance out the overuse of the left brain in the preceding decades.

Trauma survivors' need for brain integration is one reason many of us seek out a variety of creative ways, including yoga, to find this balance. Maybe someday, neuroscientists will discover that compassion also comes from a right- and left-brain integrated state. Until then, yogis already know this, perhaps especially those whose own healing depends on compassion for ourselves as well as for the causes of the trauma.

Inheriting Energy

> The body is a complex and wholly interrelated unity, fueled by food, water, air, and love and fixed by an energy field we call the spirit.
> —Hugh Milne[7]

For trauma survivors, access to our life force (prana) and awakened consciousness may occur in the process of living through the trauma itself. I have long thought that this energetic presence may originate from a "glitch" in the globe's positive energy when disaster or damage occurs. Like the fault line during an earthquake, the glitch frees up some energy that, at the point of trauma, a survivor may inherit. At the moment of impact during an accident or an explosion, when there may be fire and chaos, a person may slip out of consciousness and then emerge changed, both physically and energetically. This "glitch" can last for just a few moments and yet have a lasting impact on the rest of your life. In the case of a tsunami or earthquake this glitch can be felt in the air after such a disaster. This may be what leads people to look up at the sky, wander around quietly, kneel on the ground, and sense the world in its newness. Or, this glitch can last a long time—in the example of an attack on a village, or a police raid into a neighborhood. In the mayhem of the attack, what typically gets lost for those who survive is the chronological memory of all that occurred. The event itself was too overwhelming to comprehend at the time. What might also get lost is what is happening energetically, the rewiring at the level of the nervous system, of a community, of a way of life. This rewiring is what allows us, perhaps compels us, to see, feel, and hear the world in a new way. It is what changes us.

In my own case, early trauma was an original portal into sensing energy.[8] When I was four and my sister was two, we watched our father try to kill himself after he had gotten drunk after taking Antabuse (a drug intended to deter drinking by causing extreme negative reactions if alcohol is consumed). Powerless to his pain and screaming as he tried to pull intravenous lines out of his veins that paramedics had tried to insert while strapping him down on a gurney, part of me slipped out of my body. It was as if there was a little girl huddling with my sister in the corner of the room as well as a "see-er" looking at the whole scene from outside of myself. I might have been sensitive and a see-er before then. But the part of me that left my body could see things from an observer's position in a crystallized way—clear, open, independent, laser, original. Over the years, yoga has taught me how to sit still long enough to find that seeing power from inside myself. It is possible for me to tap into the crystalline energy that I had as a kid when I went outside of my body now without leaving my body. In fact, the adult energy now can be stronger, healthier, and more vibrant than when I was a child. This energy is connected to creativity.

This energetic awareness and heightened consciousness can give us a felt sense that is deeper than words. We can understand what the rational mind cannot—that someone is in distress even when she or he says everything is fine; that an adjustment for someone during practice that appears to be at the hip actually begins at the heart buried in grief; that the swirls of white snow you see in front of your face when you are in meditation have something to do with moving beyond a confining love relationship. It is like intuition but is more than a "gut response" since the messages can be felt in your heart and seen with your eyes.

Being able to experience the world as a "see-er" can help us heal from trauma. One step can be recalling the specific memories of how you survived. You ran away, or you reached for your sister, or you covered your head, or held your breath, or told your mother, or carried your friend to safety. Perhaps you became quiet, or you screamed bloody murder. What you did or didn't do doesn't matter as much as knowing that your response is part of the miracle of staying alive.

Another layer of healing involves uncovering the subtler, less obvious, often uncanny ways that you survived—what you acquired that you can use in the service of your own and others' healing. This level of recovery often includes finding healing energy (discovering that your hands have Reiki power, realizing you have talent as a painter, or finding yourself writing poetry, drawn to the cadence of the words).

Naming these abilities helps us see capacities we didn't know we had all those years. As it turns out, everybody has the ability to sense energy. It is what babies are doing with their big eyes before they speak, when they are taking in all the colors, shapes, textures, and feelings and then smiling back at you, toothless. Living at the level of the earth's healing energy may be what the great spiritual masters of the world—Aung San Suu Kyi, Thich Nhat Hanh, the Dalai Lama, the late Nelson Mandela, Desmond Tutu, among others—have learned to use as their guides for living. Of course, it is easy to say, "Well, I am not them; I will never be that powerful or influential." But such a comparison isn't really the point. Rather, it is coming to understand that everyone has the capacity to tap into and work with an expansive energy. This is part of what yoga practice promises.

From Iraq: Habib

Rage + confusion + grief + accountability = love
—Terry Tempest Williams[9]

At a conference on trauma, I asked the noted psychologist David Johnson why, when I tell people some of the details of sexual or physical abuse I faced, I find myself thinking that I'm making it up. I have the visual image of being sexually abused when I was still a toddler but I can't see the face, who did it to me. I know we lived in many houses when my sister and I were young, but whole slots of time and houses are missing from my memory. As I spoke, Johnson nodded in understanding and began to explain, "What we are learning from vets coming home from Iraq and Afghanistan, and from the writings about Vietnam, is that false war stories are often the ones that sound credible while true stories actually sound unbelievable, incoherent, random."[10] Fragmented memory is often a sign of truth. Stitching events together to make a coherent narrative can actually fictionalize what can only be remembered in pieces.

The inconsistency of traumatic memory is one reason that yoga can be so helpful. The practice thrives on just being on the mat, not needing to understand or solve anything. Unlike therapies that encourage people to talk about their traumatic experiences, during yoga practice there is no talking. As Sat Bir S. Khalsa, a leading yoga researcher at Harvard Medical School, explains, "With yoga . . . we don't discuss the trauma. We're interested in directly affecting the nervous system . . . making the change directly, without having to drag [trauma survivors] through it again."[11]

Trauma suffered during war and then remembered in fragments is the stuff of nightmares and flashbacks, both of which can leave people feeling unsettled. For many vets, this anxiety is longstanding, lasting years, sometimes decades. For Kevin Thames, a forty-five-year-old U.S. Army vet currently involved in a pioneering study on yoga and PTSD at the Kripalu Center for Yoga and Health in Massachusetts, problems with sleep and anger have tripped him up ever since he served in the military during Desert Storm.[12] After finding little relief in talk therapy, including that designed for those with PTSD, he signed up for the Kripalu study.

For Thames, and many others, healing involves discovering the door of a yoga studio and over time experiencing the ways that postures and meditation calm the nervous system. As Khalsa explains, unlike working out at the gym or running, "yoga works through the physical to get to the mental. We believe that in some degree [trauma] is locked up in the body. Yoga brings you right into your body, reversing that dissociation."[13] When memories that are stored in the body are released, flashbacks and nightmares may begin to diminish. Kevin Thames and other vets with PTSD are finding relief with regular yoga. Thames is sleeping better, is more focused, has lost weight, and has watched his temper diminish. Yoga is providing a peace he had not found before.

Vets are leading the way in showing us the complexity of memory and healing. In Brian Turner's *Here, Bullet,* a magnificent, chilling book of poetry based on his years as a soldier in Bosnia and then Iraq, Turner shows us that in the midst of war, the mind may only hold things that are incoherent.[14] The healing work for vets and for those who support them is to bear witness to this incoherence, knowing that it is as close to the truth as remembering may ever allow. In one of his poems, Turner writes that in Arabic, *habib* is a term of endearment that people call each other. *Habib* is what the dead speak "softly, one to another there / in the rubble and debris, *habib* / over and over, that it might not be forgotten."[15] May we all learn to whisper *habib* on and off the mat, to be witnesses, to help turn grief and confusion into love.

Walking Meditation and the Great Migration

And now the teaching on yoga begins.
Yoga is the settling of the mind into silence.
　　—Patanjali[16]

Many people who have just started coming to yoga find that "settling of the mind into silence" is difficult. Very difficult. You may be able to land a headstand (sirsasana) within the first three months, hold tree pose *(vrksasana)* as if you were an oak in another life, and go from a deep lunge into a full split *(hanumanasana),* but when it comes to sitting in silence, just plain sitting, you might feel like you must run immediately right out of the room. Meditation (dhyana) is a not such an easy task for people who have been putting out fires since we were little; who jump at the sound of any loud noise; who are afraid to close our eyes at night, never mind during the day; who have a hard time finding breath. That's okay. That's normal. The mat can take your impatience. We are not alone.

My friend and fellow yoga practitioner Diane has had a hard time sitting still most of her life. In first grade the teacher tied her to her desk, telling her if she didn't learn how to sit still she wouldn't be allowed to come to school again. A willful and smart child, she had already been skipped out of kindergarten. As one of the only children in the neighborhood whose family had a whole set of encyclopedias, she had developed a real curiosity for learning. But when it came to keeping her body quiet, she found little success. Childhood was like that for her, a lot getting in the way of being still. When she was still in her crib, Diane had an asthma attack that left her desperately gasping for air, no adults around to help her. She remembers thrashing about, petrified that she could not get enough air in her body. Since then, the idea of sitting still and focusing entirely on her breath brought her back to that panic and aloneness. As a child, Diane also did whatever she could to leave her house—a place of sadness, drinking, and mental illness—feeling much safer outside with the chickens, the trees, the neighbors.

As an adult, her multiple attempts to sit in meditation at the beginning or end of a yoga practice left her feeling more agitated than when she began, a reality that eventually led her to decide that when it came to meditation, she was a failure. It wasn't until she attended a workshop for faculty bringing contemplative practices into their classrooms that she found a way to meditate that worked for her. In this workshop, facilitator Maribai Bush instructed the class that for the morning session, they could either meditate by sitting together in silence, or walk in meditation outdoors. Diane was thrilled. As she slowly walked on the grounds of the retreat center saying the mantra "I am walking, I am here, I am home," she relaxed in a way she never had when sitting. She was amused that it made her so happy, calling me that afternoon to report to me she was no longer a failed meditator. She said, "All this sitting still waiting for something to happen was too hard for me. This was easy." For Diane, the walking meditation was similar to drawing in her coloring book, a meditation she had begun doing in her forties, often after teaching her college classes or attending faculty meetings. She found the movement of her hand on the page calming. Choosing colors and staying between the lines helped quiet her mind and gave her the focus she needed to be still.

A few years after discovering walking meditation, Diane came across Yoga Nidra, a practice that encourages deep relaxation where the mind rests between wakefulness and dreaming. As was true for the walking meditation, with Yoga Nidra, Diane had something to concentrate on beyond the breath—in this instance the instructor's voice—as she was guided to send breath to her toes, ankles, knees, hips, and up her body. Diane became so proficient at this type of meditation that now she can do it in the bathtub by herself. Instead of thinking of nothing (as she associates with still meditation) she can move the water around her body while getting into a state that feels like being asleep. She uses the physical sensation of the water moving to go along with the focus in order to relax.

What asthma taught Diane is that even when she was very little, there was a connection between the mind and breath. Her concentration on getting enough oxygen in her body kept her alive. This experience let her know that concentration and meditation are capacities that reside within us. They aren't external abilities that we need to learn from others. It took her years to understand that she was seeking what she already knew. Asthma had corrupted her relationship to meditation, by making it an anxious relationship associated with a fear of dying.[17] The walking meditation and Yoga Nidra helped her get in touch with the focus she had as a three-year-old. Without the fear of stillness, she could focus on movement, a human voice, warm water.

While Diane's story is a uniquely individual one—a little girl with asthma growing up in Iowa who, as an adult, discovers walking meditation—her story has communal resonance as well. As an African American woman growing up in the twentieth century, Diane comes from a long line of people who could not stay still, who had to keep moving as a response to the trauma of slavery. On her mother's side of the family, people ran from the South to Oklahoma and Kansas, changing names and racial designations on more than one occasion. Her father's side of the family left the South for all points west as well. There is a deep strain of running from trauma in Diane's bones and blood. A deep strain of not sitting still. Yoga Nidra and walking meditation have been part of her journey in understanding these ancestral connections, of honoring those who have chosen freedom over enslavement, sometimes having to gasp for breath along the way.

Between Heroin and a Headstand

> When I first started teaching yoga, I wasn't leading a so-called yoga lifestyle, although I was practicing occasionally and teaching. I was actually leading two lives. I was still doing drugs intermittently. I was still feeling depressed. I was not caring for myself in good ways, although I was trying to.
> —Patricia Walden[18]

A stumbling block that some people experience to getting to the mat is facing the contradiction between what our lives look like and what we think they should look like. Many of us have idealized versions of what it means to be a yoga practitioner, to have a regular practice . . . versions that can keep us from being honest about the contradictions we live with, the paradoxes we often don't have language to explain.

This is one reason why, when I first read an interview with Patricia Walden, one of the most revered Iyengar teachers in the United States, I felt so much respect for her. In the interview she writes about her path from heroin addiction and surviving a grueling childhood, telling brave truths about how yoga began for her as a means of self-soothing. She explains that in her early years of yoga, "there was a big gap between my inner life and my outer life, so I felt like a fake much of the time. It is agonizing when you're going to a class and teaching yoga and you know you're not living it a hundred percent even though you believe in it."[19] This disjuncture is what led her to take seriously the injuries she had faced as a child. She started to understand that she hadn't been using heroin to party but rather to self-medicate.

For Walden, a big step away from addictions and other harmful behavior came from recognizing the strengths she had to develop in order to survive. She writes, "I think that most kids who grow up in dysfunctional families like mine feel very alone. You have to figure things out for yourself: how to nurture yourself, how to take care of yourself. It has some benefits, of course. As a result of my experience, I'm a survivor."[20] From this naming, this honesty, this breaking of silences can come beginning steps in making new choices. As her practice deepened, she began to ask herself, "Ok, if I do this drug, how am I going to feel a week from now? On the other hand, if I go to my mat and do Headstand, how am I going to feel a week from now? . . . It is so powerful, that little moment of freedom and grace where for whatever reason you are able to pause before making your decision."[21]

In these and so many other instances, freedom is not some grandiose state that comes after your graduate, retire, die. Freedom is not restricted to those who can find enlightenment from studying a wall for years at a time. Freedom starts with being willing to choose between doing heroin and a headstand. It starts with moving your way through the contradictions that make you human.

Inside Silence

My world has changed its shape tonight. A new level of me is coming alive. I am overwhelmed with the feeling that my body has been waiting for me to stop neglecting it, waiting for me to quiet down and listen.

—Matthew Sanford[22]

Many trauma survivors who come to yoga discover that paying attention to the subtle sensations in our bodies is key to learning to listen to them. For Matthew Sanford, a yoga instructor and writer who survived a car accident when he was thirteen years old, finding yoga in his twenties taught him to pay attention to sensations in his body that he had been taught to ignore. Sanford lost his father and sister in the accident, and he was paralyzed from the chest down. In the process of recovery, Sanford endured living inside a halo (which actually required the insertion of screws into his head), multiple surgeries, several body casts, and years of physical therapy. Along the way, he was taught what he called a "medical healing story" from many doctors and physical therapists that led him to dismiss the sensations he often still felt in his legs as phantom and to believe that his legs were essentially dead.

Ten years later, through a combination of his own inquisitiveness and grace, he met an Iyengar yoga instructor, whose precise attention to alignment and gifts of intuition helped him reconnect with sensations and an energetic awareness of his legs. Sanford describes the moment when this first happened during a session with his teacher when she showed him *maha mudra* (a seated pose where one leg is straight and the other is bent with the sole of the foot on the inner thigh, the fingers of both hands are linked to the outstretched big toe, and the abdomen is pulled toward the spine). All of a sudden, Sanford experienced "a new *ding*. I suddenly feel a tangible sense of my whole body—inside and out, paralyzed and unparalyzed. I am stunned."[23] Along with this breakthrough came a deeper understanding about the multiple meanings of silence. The silence that Sanford experienced in his body when he was paralyzed stayed with him all those years.

For many years Sanford had interpreted the silence as deadness in his limbs. He writes, "When those screws were twisted into my thirteen-year-old head, my existence was spread so thin that a sinewy silence was revealed, a silence that coexisted with my living, a silence that made me stronger. It was my death."[24] With time he learned to experience the silence as a quiet that enabled him to find sensations such as buzzing, tingling, and humming. When a person's legs are fully functional, they give messages at a high decibel. If you are paralyzed, the messages are subtler. Through yoga Sanford learned that silence has many registers and that it is possible to become attuned to them. This awareness allowed him to reconnect with the parts of his body that he had been told to give up on.

Yoga has not helped him walk again, but Sanford can do an exciting range of yoga postures. And, perhaps more importantly, he has an awareness of his entire body, along with access to emotions and a faith in his body that he thought had died during the accident. As Sanford discovered, "mind-body integration is not just a personal health strategy, it is a potentially evolutionary movement of consciousness."[25]

Many trauma survivors have had to confront the possibility of dying. But the silence that a person associates with death may be a guide to discovering the body again. Sitting with that silence can move a person from no memory of an event—a blank spot suspended in fog—to discovering gifts from a brave healing path. The mind-body integration that Sanford was finding through practicing carefully aligned postures enabled him to start having flashbacks about the accident. These flashbacks led to dreams where his sister who had died in the accident held him. He had an encounter with his near death experience following the accident, and he befriended the vulnerable, feminine aspects of his consciousness he had been asked to put aside after the accident. As he absorbed the death of the young boy who could walk, he confronted the medical protocol that asked him to leave his body behind. As he used yoga to return to his body, he committed to living fully, recognizing birth and death as inextricably related.

"At Birth We Know Everything"

At birth we know everything, can see into the shimmer of complexity. When a newborn looks at you it is with utter comprehension. We know where we are coming from, where we have been. And then we forget it all. That's why infants sleep so much after birth. It is an adjustment.

—Joy Harjo[26]

Several months after coming to one of my classes, a man in his fifties, a vet, asked me why, at the end of so many practices, I suggest that people roll to the right and curl up in a fetal position before slowly sitting up for meditation. As we talked, we came to surmise that, perhaps, each practice can be understood as a little birth, symbolized in the fetal position as well as a little death (of old patterns, bad moods, loneliness). Yoga gives us a chance to know what we knew as newborns, the expansiveness of life. This is what people mean by "beginner's mind"—coming to the mat each day as if it is our first.

Beginning to heal through yoga includes remembering what you knew, felt, and loved before danger and fears moved in. Writing about her capacious awareness as a child, yogi Konda Mason writes, "Often I would fill up with so much joy that I would turn into particles of energy hovering above my bed. I would buzz around like a firefly in small packets of light energy. I remember an amazing feeling of expansion and connection."[27] Mason was able to tap into this experience in a daily way, knowing that it had something to do with "God and me as One." When she was twelve, however, when her family moved to a white suburb, her connection to the unlimited was severed. She writes that as an African American girl, "the dualistic world of 'us' and 'them' forced its way into my life and psyche. I could no longer find the 'One.' I spent my teenage years longing for some way to reconcile with this world filled with hatred and bigotry, as the racism in America and the war in Vietnam raged on."[28]

For Mason, yoga led her back to the consciousness she had before racism intervened. She writes, "As I lay in *savasana* . . . I began to relive the experience of that expanded consciousness I had felt as a child. My heart opened wide. As I sat in meditation I felt my connection to all beings. The compassion within me swelled. It was as if the sound of the birds and the scent of night-blooming jasmine had come back. I was home again."[29] Yoga can be like that, coming home again, beginning to "see into the shimmer of complexity," one posture at a time.

"Common Ground Is We"

Common ground
is we, forever
breathing this earth
—Sonia Sanchez[30]

When I first started yoga, I did everything I could to follow the teacher's instructions. Raised by a mother who was a gifted teacher, I automatically brought respect for the instructor to class. How that translated for me was hurting my back, fairly significantly, pushing to get into dancer pose (*dandayamana dhanurasana*) and seated forward bend (*paschimottanasana*) way before my lower back was open enough. It took having to take a few months off from yoga and all exercise (which in my life felt like an eternity) to realize that my first guide needs to be my body, the second (and a distant one) the instructor.

This lesson can be an especially hard one for survivors to accept, our hope to find people we can trust and who will take care of us seemingly insatiable. To back off and have to listen to my body first felt like defeat, lonely and embarrassing. And yet, the Yoga Sutras tell us that yoga is about finding comfort and ease in the pose—not someone else's picture-perfect pose but our own. The promise, then, is not to be photographed for the cover of *Yoga Journal* or deemed ready to move to the advanced class, or admired for our agility, athletic prowess. The promise is those irreplaceable milli-moments of awareness, steadiness, connection.

These milli-moments of awareness made me think about how certain poses can feel like haiku poems—a poetic form that manages to say in seventeen syllables what might take whole books and lifetimes to say otherwise—simple, compact nuggets of awareness that can come from being honest with ourselves, listening to our bodies. For trauma survivors, one reason to pay attention to alignment and then adjust accordingly is that the postures are like safe containers. Each has its own parameters, its own boundaries that we learn to work with based on our own anatomy. I am remembering how, the first time I did pigeon pose (eka pada raja kapotasana) with my forward knee more bent, rather than how I had been taught (with my calf perpendicular to my thigh), I could then really settle in on top of my legs, and swan bow to the ground feeling a sense of humility and grace at the same time. Like I had come home somehow. Pigeon pose becomes "common ground // is we, forever // breathing this earth."

At the Risk of Unraveling

When Rosie first came to yoga class she informed me that her body was so tight she was afraid she might simply snap if she started to stretch. During the first class, she set her mat right next to mine, and proceeded to moan throughout the entire practice, letting all of us know that something, seemingly everything, hurt. After practice, as people milled around, Rosie approached me and asked if I would massage her shoulders, having noticed that I had done so for another practitioner. I remember feeling surprised that she would be so assertive after her very first time in my class. I was heartened, though, that she wasn't afraid to ask for what she needed.

Once everyone had left and the shoulder massage had ended, she told me that her body had been hurting for several years, ever since her partner had beaten her. While the abuse was over, she said his beatings had left their mark—a seemingly permanent ache in her shoulders and neck. She told me that she had been looking for something like this class for years, and was grateful to have finally found it. Afterward, she came regularly for a few months. She didn't mention our initial conversation again but always set her mat up in the same place, right next to mine.

Then she disappeared. When I called her and left a message saying I missed seeing her, she didn't return my call. Eventually she did come back, arriving for class at the very last moment, setting up her mat in the back of the room, and leaving as soon as we were done, never meeting my eyes. This continued until a few months later, when a new teacher came to my class to assist. Rosie reached out to the teacher after class, asking for a shoulder rub, and then telling her the same history she had told me, almost verbatim, with the same urgency and immediacy. As she had done with me, she said how much she appreciated the yoga, and reiterated her intention to come often.

And then, just as had happened before, her attendance became intermittent, until finally it ended. Perhaps she will return. Or not. Perhaps she will find other yoga classes. Or not.

The stepping in, stepping out, the move toward contact, followed by the pulling away, makes a lot of sense for trauma survivors. You find something that feels good, you feel seen and acknowledged, but then you get scared, apprehensive about having to sustain contact over time.

This is early yoga for many. Two steps in, one step out. Connect to a new face, then retreat to safer ground.

Bam!

I am out to dinner with two of my friends, both women in the prime of their lives (in their sixties) who have been practicing yoga since their teens. They are both writers and seasoned yoga teachers who turn heads wherever we go, their dreads, braids, stylish dress, sexy bodies landing us the best booth at the restaurant, an especially attentive waitress, guaranteed great conversation through the vegetarian meal. Over dessert I ask them how yoga has changed them, what they might say that they haven't seen written about elsewhere, that is unique to their own stories. The birthday woman, Wyoma, starts out, "I come from a religious clan of people, knowing when I was young that I needed to leave that system, step out of the church, which I did at fifteen, except for the choir, which I stayed in, always loving the music. I left still hungry for spirituality, wondering if it is possible to satisfy that hunger without religion. Then I fell into yoga, finding a book that I read on the spot, and bam! I knew my life was changed, have never turned back, forty-five years later. Yoga has been my door and doorway."[31]

My other friend, Anna Dunwell, nodding her way through Wyoma's "bam story," says, "Well, at the risk of sounding dramatic, I would say that yoga saved my life. You see, there is this story in the Bible that it is difficult for a rich man to go through the eye of a needle. Well I was that man—I had it all—money, riches, freedom. I was married to a white man who was making six figures, we had a fancy house and five people who were taking care of my every need. As many around me looked on in shock, shaking their heads, I left with my two-and-a-half-year-old daughter, walked out of that American dream, knowing I needed to reinhabit my own life, my own body—a process that led me straight into yoga, where I have been since. That is what yoga can do, make it possible to go through the eye of a needle, leave what is stopping such a journey."[32]

That is the thing about yoga; it can catch you early or catch you late. It can keep you company when you walk out on the husband everyone thinks is the one for you or give you a spiritual life the church cannot fill. And, if your life is anything like these two women's—full of gifts and struggles, sending them both trauma and healing—then yoga gets to be the transitional object, what you can come back to over time.

Rapture

As many of the entries in this first section attest, when people who have faced loss or betrayal first come to yoga, it can be scary—with emotions, memories, sensations, pain coming up that you didn't expect, that you had perhaps tried to protect yourself from for a long time, maybe years. But early yoga is also about feeling joy. That is what gets people to bring their friends for the first time and what keeps people coming back.

I'm thinking, for example, of a recent class where, well into the practice, I looked around to see Brenda—an ex-military woman with a thousand jeweled braids who had been coming to yoga regularly for several months—with an expression on her face that can only be described as rapture. We had been practicing for about forty minutes—had made it through several energizing postures, including the breath of joy; had done balancing sequences in a circle, holding on to each other to make a collective wreath as each of us landed the pose.[33] We had done garland *(malasana),* squatting together and then rocking back and forth while some people eased their way into crow (bakasana), balancing on their triceps, while others shook their heads, using that pose as a reason to do child's pose (balasana). One person announced "I got it, I got it," while another shook her head in awe, a third staying with the rock, back and forth, back and forth, grinning. We were definitely doing a lot of laughing. Everyone had walked downward-facing dog *(adho mukha svanasana)* around the room, their derrieres pointed up to the sky, lifting their heads whenever they were about to bump into someone else. Luther Vandross had carried us through an undulating Sun Salutation series (surya namaskar) and Patti LaBelle had helped us through pyramid sway *(prasarita padottanasana)* while finger painting on the ground. This sequence of poses, especially with the delightful, eclectic, intergenerational, all-kinds-of-bodies-in-the-room crowd that had come that day, was enough to manufacture some joy.

But I think what really put the practice over the top was the young couple, in their twenties, with their Rastafarian hats and carefully designed tattoos, who had brought the woman's mother with them. This was her first time to yoga, an elderly woman who was struggling to get up and down, who clearly was facing a number of physical limitations and, I am guessing, had seen a lot in her life, not all of it pretty. Regardless, she had spent the practice trying, really trying. And you could tell that she could feel the love in the room. In a way, it didn't matter whether she could walk her dog or raise her arms above her head. What mattered was that her daughter and son-in-law brought her, understanding yoga as a physical and spiritual practice that has been, can be, intergenerational.

This is, I am guessing, part of what Brenda was picking up on. And maybe, too, she was noticing my glistening eyes since people knew that this was the last day we were all going to be together for two months (as I was on my way to teach yoga in Thailand). Halfway through practice, as we held each other's arms up to the sky, all of us in various stages of tree pose in a circle (vrksasana turned into a forest), I got such an overwhelming burst of elation that it felt like someone had turned the music up on life and kept it cranked up high.[34] Then I looked over, as we were moving from raising our hands toward the sky and then cascading toward the ground while sitting kneeling in a circle, and I saw Brenda's face, as each reach to the sky brought gratitude and joy through her body. It was as if she was praying with a yoga sway—a combination of the music, the good-bye day, the intergenerational attendance, the collective movement—bringing the spirit into the room.

This is what early yoga can be like: Brenda, announcing at the beginning of class that "I've been coming for a bit now, trying never to miss a class," welcoming an elder, showing the new young ones how it can be done, bringing her love of living right into the center of the practice. All of us feeling the music. All of us together. In that moment, no trauma, no injury, no barrier, no fear. Just there, enjoying.

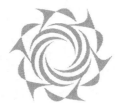

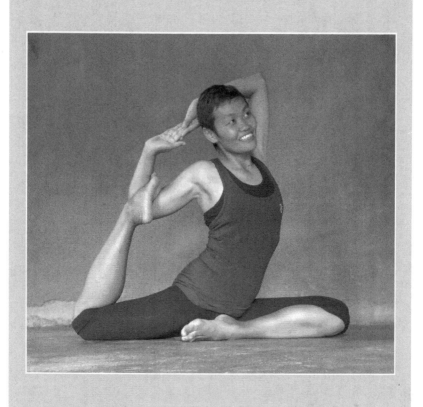

PART II

Like Dragonflies

What Makes Trauma Survivors Special

Hands without irons become dragonflies,
red flowers rain on our hats,
subversive angels flutter like pigeons from a rooftop,
this stripped and starving earth is not a grave.
　　—Martín Espada[1]

One day, in the midst of planning a workshop on trauma for yoga instructors, I realized I had hit my limit in talking about the challenges and extra work that trauma survivors require. I was weary of the litany of common guidelines for how to work with trauma survivors: use a soothing voice, always ask if you can touch before doing an assist; always require consent forms so that if someone has a negative reaction during practice you are covered.

It's not that any of this wasn't valid. Working with trauma survivors can be intense. We survivors may need quiet voices, extra time. We may be quirky, and have difficulty following rote directions. We may have flashbacks, dissociate. While in many ways I am grateful for the research of the last decade, which has put the subject of trauma on the national radar and created a new level of sensitivity toward survivors, this work can become doctrinaire. Creating a template with a whole set of guidelines, trainings, and protocols to use in working with survivors runs the risk of putting the emphasis on what is wrong with survivors, lumping us all into a category of subjects that needs to be studied, spoken for, and fixed.

What may go missing from this work is recognition that survivors also embody many strengths—qualities that are worth noting, paying attention to, and even celebrating. That is what inspired the entries in "Like Dragonflies" and why this section opens with an idiosyncratic, anecdotal, and hopefully helpful list of what makes survivors special.

Understanding trauma survivors starts with knowing the conditions that created the pain we have experienced. Survivors are not, as individuals, the problem. Using war to resolve human conflicts is the problem, not the war veterans themselves. Sexual violation of children is the problem, not the children themselves. Survivors are the canaries in the coal mine, not the poisonous gas that kills the miners. Survivors have been figuring out ways to overcome post–traumatic stress disorder for years, long before the Department of Defense began spending money on programs for returning vets. Granted, there are therapists, doctors, and yoga instructors who are trauma specialists, but those who survived trauma will always be the experts.

A number of people whose stories appear in this section see the process of healing as a journey that is as much spiritual as physical or psychological. They believe that in the course of healing they have gained access to spiritual capacities that should be recognized and supported. The scholar and poet Akasha Gloria Hull tells us that those who live through the isolation and injury resulting from emotional or sexual abuse often develop a rich interior life when young.[2] They are the kids reading Kafka as teenagers, taking themselves to church or synagogue because that is where they can find real discussion of suffering, the meaning of life. They may be the poets, the odd ones whose noses are buried in books when holidays devolve into orgies of food and drink. The same can be said for adults who live through trauma who often create original and innovative methods for healing on and off the mat.

Survivors have a lot to teach. For example, many have access to what is referred to, in meditation and yoga circles, as witnessing, which is the ability to step out of one's immediate circumstances—out of a conflict at work, a self-negating inner dialogue, a stuck place between two lovers—and see it from a more detached place.

Trauma survivors also understand compassion, not just for themselves but for those who injured them. If we really listen to trauma survivors, we learn a lot about what we need to know about compassion, that silky, illusive softness that develops when forgiveness is in the room, when rage is slowly replaced by understanding, by letting go.

Leading with compassion and respect does wonders for everybody, perhaps especially for survivors of trauma, who are much more likely to be receptive to suggestions if they first feel recognized for who they are, for what it took to make it alive out of the bedroom, the alleyway, the war zone, or the hurricane. Survivors are more likely to stay on the mat, reach deeper into a pose, try a headstand, be able to hear the teacher if they are first seen for what makes them distinct, unique, and brave.

This is why, when I am asked to assist in a teacher training, I often find myself down on all fours whispering to someone in child's pose (balasana) or shoulder stand *(sarvangasana)*, "You have a beautiful practice," or "You have such presence on the mat."

This is what I have been learning from survivors. Start with what we are doing well. Start with what makes us special. We are all walking miracles. If a yoga studio is set up to see survivors, really acknowledge them, it will be set up to see everyone. That is how it works.

That is how we work—subversive missionaries on the road to health.

Survivor Strengths

> I believe that by changing ourselves we change the world, that traveling El Mundo Zurdo path is the path of a two-way movement—a going deep into the self and an expanding out into the world, a simultaneous re-creation of the self and a reconstruction of society.
>
> —Gloria Anzaldúa[3]

Sometimes when the phrase *trauma survivor* is mentioned, there is such heaviness in the air, such hesitation and deliberate conversation that I just want to shout—"Don't be afraid of survivors; don't back away. They might be you and you might be them." So instead of starting with what is challenging, stressful, and complicated about working with survivors, I want to celebrate our strengths:

- Survivors do much emotional, physical, spiritual, and mental work to stay in the world, to be present. That takes guts.

- Many survivors need to talk about what we feel, think, experience, are surprised by, and learn. Many of us need regular conversation about what is going on, what it takes to be fully present. So does everyone. Imagine if we made time for that kind of intimacy in our everyday lives.

- People who have lived through trauma often strike me as a kind of left-handed people, living in what Chicana theorist Gloria Anzaldúa calls *"el mundo zurdo"* (a left-handed world).[4] People who live a left-handed life bring originality to yoga classes. Who wants a yoga class where everyone is doing postures exactly the same, coming in and out of poses on the same breath, able to fling themselves into all kinds of postures without much struggle? The most interesting classes are often the quirky ones, where people's responses are unique, unexpected, surprising. You can often count on survivors to bring that left-handed reality to classes.

- The hypervigilance that many survivors have makes us a particularly stimulating bunch. Another, more positive way we might talk about hypervigilance is having a heightened awareness, a self-consciousness that creates a certain kind of insight and sensitivity. It is as if survivors have an additional chamber of consciousness. We are always watching on many levels, every day Geiger counters for what is going on.

• Many survivors are really good listeners. They bring this ability to the yoga studio. They are ones you can count on not to talk over other people's experiences, who know that being a witness for people does not necessarily mean filling the space with talk. In fact, sometimes just the opposite is crucial—sitting, with no words, all compassion.

• Survivors often recognize others in distress. That is why we can get exhausted, because our sensors are always on. In yoga classes we can be helpful not only to fellow canaries but for other birds as well—wrens, hummingbirds, storks, even kiwis.

• Survivors on a healing path are often gifted healers as well. Having lived through an experience can make all the difference in deeply connecting with others who have struggled. In his gorgeous book, *The Heart of Listening,* about the spiritual and energetic journey for craniosacral therapists, Hugh Milne writes, "I have known many therapists, many healers. . . . It is quite apparent to me that the more chaotic the individual's personal life has been, the more gifted a therapist she becomes. The more pain she has suffered and transcended, the deeper her love and the more supportive her compassion."[5] There is nothing like the humility and tenderness that comes from living through tragedy or loss to help people know empathy from the inside out, from deep inside.

• Survivors are often at the center of building creative communities—yoga studios with sliding fee scales; yoga classes for people with HIV; meditation classes for genocide survivors; yoga for children and their parents. With trauma, the invulnerability that people may carry with them before they were raped, before they lose a parent to a sudden accident, or before they witness police brutality gets replaced with the knowledge that the world can be dangerous. Trauma survivors know, from experience, that the ground is shaking for many people. That direct knowledge clicks many of us into gear. Makes us activists. Requires us to build communities that can sustain us.

• We may see the world more rather than less accurately than the less traumatized—we have had to.[6] This worldview doesn't mean we don't have to deal with our own distortions, fears, flashbacks, etc. But when you check out those who are making justice in your communities, chances are they have seen trauma.

• We have a way of keeping hope alive even when that might seem like too much to ask. Recently, I asked my housemate, Desmond, who has been through his share of struggles (including many years living on a shoestring and a mental health issue that took a long time to diagnose), what he would say about trauma survivors. First laughing at my question, he then offered a story with his Jamaican lilt coming through as he spoke. "I was sitting by one of my kindergarten students today who tells me with her small voice that her life is difficult. All of my life experience tells me to say to her, 'You can overcome anything, even if it is really hard. You can do it.' It is the meditation and yoga I do that takes me to the place of knowing that there is hope, for her and for me."

We gravitate toward each other and then build a community of healers by setting up ongoing dialogues. We are special because where there is pain, there is hope. Meditation and yoga teach us that we don't have to always experience that pain, especially when we stretch together—and listen.

Object Permanence on the Mat

Sometimes when I am taking a Bikram yoga class, where we do the same twenty-six postures and two breathing exercises, in exactly the same order, I often ask myself questions: "How can you possibly think it is helpful to practice the same postures day after day? Are you scared of classes that have more variety? Maybe you're stuck. Plenty of people think Bikram yoga is too rigid. What's up with you?"

Fortunately, a kinder voice intervenes, one that I have spent years cultivating (not always with success) that reminds me that many people have faced the same dilemma. Rolf Gates writes that many people come to yoga feeling that something is missing. This feeling "manifests in a desire for more: more yoga postures, harder yoga postures, more classes per week, more workshops, more teachers." Gates suggests that this restlessness can actually be a useful indicator, that what "we need is not to dig a new well, but to dig even more deeply the well we are already in."[7] And it is true: there is something about practicing the same twenty-six postures that lets me go deeper rather than wider, slows me down.

This repetitive practice might be especially helpful for those who didn't experience what developmental psychologists refer to as "object permanence" when we were very young (infancy to two years old). Object permanence is the ability to know that objects and people—like your dad!—still exist even when you can't see them. Infants and toddlers who are in the process of mastering this developmental milestone laugh over and over again when someone keeps ducking around a corner and then pops out again a moment later, surprising them each time this reappearance occurs. Peekaboo is actually a profound lesson in phenomenology. Before mastering that lesson, the child is unable to conceptualize that something that is visually absent has not permanently disappeared.

Adults who missed this developmental process may have a hard time believing that if someone leaves you, even briefly—to go to work, on a trip, or even out to dinner with someone else—that that person will return. In my own life, I have surmised that a combination of my father's intermittent presence (as a parent who cuddled and held me) and how difficult it was for my teen mother to be consistently present meant I didn't develop object permanence. As an adult this missing ability manifested itself in several ways, including realizing that if my long-term lover was far away, I automatically assumed that she was dead. "You're still alive," I would think in shock the first moment I heard her voice on the phone—before my conscious mind could remind me that of course she was alive, and doing good work in some other part of the world. It took years of her leaving and coming back before I started to trust, in my deepest, unconscious self, that if she left, she would eventually return.

Many trauma survivors either had no opportunity to experience object permanence in our earliest years, or had later experiences of losing loved ones that shattered a sense of permanence. For me, object permanence as it relates to people has had to develop alongside my ability to see my own body as permanent. This too is a challenge for many people, who lost a sense of their bodies as their own. Their bodies were lent to others, borrowed by others, stolen. How this relates to yoga is that for them the act of doing the same postures over and over—rather than practicing new postures or finding new yoga teachers—can be a lesson in permanence. It tells them that they are real, and their bodies are real, which is a huge step toward knowing that those they love are real too, and that they will come back.

Nowadays, I would describe myself as a yoga polygamist. I practice as well as teach from an eclectic palette of traditions. But the minute things feel shaky in my life I am back on the Bikram mat, in the same place in the studio, doing those same postures in the same early morning class, with the same loyalist yogis who go to that class—trying to listen to my body, to hear the familiar anthems it has sung so many times before. This is comfort. This, it turns out, gives me strength.

Dancing the Tango

Several years ago one of my teachers told me that the work of trauma survivors is to create new memory—an assertion that left me perplexed. As I was diligently trying to create some sort of coherent narrative about my childhood that rang true for me, the idea that I could choose to tell the story in another way felt scary—made it seem like truth was so relative that I didn't know how I could trust it. But over time I have come to see that my teacher was talking about how memory is a living and breathing entity. For example, accepting that my sister and I lived with our fear button on automatic (in response to punishment, violence, and constant uprooting) allowed me to also marvel at our deep love for each other, our creative resilience. Alongside my averted gaze in photos, the bald spots on my sister's and my heads from a parent pulling our hair out, were two inseparable towheads climbing trees like they were couches, making the boys in the neighborhood run if they tried anything nasty. The more I am willing to get inside of poses during practice and welcome into consciousness what before was buried, the more three-dimensional the story about my life becomes.

I am not saying that now, if I had a chance to choose whether I experienced childhood trauma or not, I would say yes. I take issue with the notion that everything has a reason. But trauma does open ways of being in the world, a questioning, vulnerable, constant growing spirit that makes us who we are. The steps of healing require us to get to know and eventually integrate into our lives the irregularities we have experienced. Over time we break these irregularities into bite-size pieces until we can incorporate them into a larger frame.

A great analogy I have found for the process that trauma survivors go through in healing is embedded in the language used to teach people the tango. In a recent tango class, the irreverent teacher explained that tango can be understood as a grammar of moves.[8] It is made up of a number of regular (predictable) steps as well as irregular steps, what in linguistics would be called "idioms." He defined idioms as "assimilable irregularities"—patterns of steps that we make sense of through their peculiarity that, over time, become an integral part of the dance. In tango, the first assimilable irregularity is called the *salida,* which opens the dance with a four-step beat that looks like a three step beat.[9] The salida is essential to the dance—in fact, the dance could not begin without it. It is hard to imagine dance and language without idioms, these assimilable irregularities that have woven themselves into the fabric of our cultural art forms.

Learning how to tango sounds like healing from trauma. Injuries that, at the time they occur, are unassimilable, but then can, eventually, become assimilated. They get woven into the narratives we create about our lives. To me, one of the most mysterious and remarkable aspects of the body is its ability to hold trauma in its unassimilable form until we have the resources and support we need to bring it to consciousness. That is what yoga does—it gives us the resources to deal with the pain that is stored in the body. The gentleness of the mat and the consistency of the practice open a way for us to move through pain without getting snagged. This movement has the potential to transform memories from irregularities that remain on an unconscious level to ones we can pull into consciousness—to make them part of our speech, our known reality, a pattern to work with and change. Asanas and breath work can help us make trauma an "assimilable irregularity" that gives us personality, perseverance, and purpose along the way. There is a way out (a salida) from trauma that also means the beginning of our own original dance.

Like a Homily

One of the lessons that survivors have to teach us is the ingenious ways they find to cope with trauma. A powerful example of this can be seen in the life of a yogi friend of mine, John Brown, a fifty-year-old father, husband, veteran, and police detective of African American and Cherokee descent who considers yoga the best way he has found to deal with the stresses life has brought his direction. When he started practicing yoga five years ago, he had a terrible time sleeping, had been taking medication for chronic acid reflux for years, was carrying around extra weight, and was constantly anxious. He developed these PTSD symptoms when he was in the Marines, in particular from the period during Desert Storm. When he was in the military, he learned how to keep emotions at bay because he had to get ready for the next mission. His unit was engaged in heavy combat on the "Highway of Death" in Iraq and on other reconnaissance missions. He tells me, "That death and fear and stress stays in the body. We never got any training about how to deal with that before we went or after. We brought that back to our families and communities."

Soon after returning, John became a sergeant in the homicide unit of the Boston Police Department. He began to see that the stresses of the job did little to combat his symptoms. With each murder he investigates, the media demands graphic details for their stories, authorities downtown want immediate answers, and people in neighborhoods understandably are distraught seeing dead bodies in their communities. Of all the stresses, seeing what the families of those who have been murdered go through weighs on John the most. John and his coworkers do all they can so that some sort of dignity is left to the person who has died, as well as for their families. John admits, "It is a very heavy burden. I get completely involved with the families. This job has a long tail. It never goes away."

Two years into the job, a detective buddy dragged John to a yoga class. As someone who was muscle-bound, well over two hundred pounds, and six-foot-three, John felt like "an elephant, lumbering and out of balance." He felt like he couldn't breathe, had to use the wall during standing poses, couldn't keep his elbows up during the opening breathing exercise, and couldn't reach his ankles. He found it impossible to put any weight on his knees for camel (ustrasana), and he had trouble absorbing the dialogue. While he might follow the cues for the first few postures, pretty soon he would tune out the words, flailing about just to try to make it through the series. He quickly discovered that what he thought was a feminine, lightweight practice was actually intense and demanding. He started to notice he could sleep soundly in a bed after years of sleeping sitting up. And he was finding a calm at work that he didn't know was possible. He found himself going straight to practice right after working a night shift, finding it the best way to wind down.

Over time, he saw that the physical benefits from yoga were coupled with emotional growth. Before he started yoga he struggled with impatience. He explained to me, "In war, if people can't keep up, if they are not 'wired up tight,' they can get killed. We can all get killed. I was part of a small unit. We absolutely needed to depend on each other. It has taken a lot for me to understand that sometimes I don't need that hypervigilance now, that my impatience is not always useful. Yoga demands a tremendous amount of patience."

John is also seeing that symptoms associated with PTSD can be turned into strengths. The hypervigilance he developed during Desert Storm also gives him remarkable abilities to sort through evidence and remember detail. His ingenuity is in learning how to channel that hyperalertness, and to let it go when he doesn't need it. Recently, John applied these skills when he was the lead detective for a quadruple homicide case. It was one of the most gruesome murder cases in Boston history, involving the death of a two-year-old child, his mother, and two other people. The trial was complicated and contested. For five days straight, John was on the stand. He watched as the techniques he worked on in yoga—being present on the mat, being able to hold his concentration, keeping his chin and chest up so that he could breathe deeply—were vital to practice on the stand. As it turns out, when the trial began, John was in the middle of a fifty-day challenge (one class a day for fifty days) in concert with his fiftieth birthday. The challenge helped him usher in his birthday as he listened deeply and stayed focused through the trial.

His disciplined practice also kept him focused on changing his eating patterns that resulted in losing sixty-five pounds. For years, he would go all day without eating and then gorge himself at night. He survived on coffee, pizza, and subs. Since he started eating six small meals instead, beginning with breakfast, the weight has been steadily declining. The owner of the yoga studio says that she can't recognize him now. "I don't look like the same person. I can do every posture. I never need the wall. I feel very strong." And he never takes the little purple pill, Prilosec for acid reflux, that he took for over a decade. He has also witnessed a dramatic change in his drinking. Before yoga, he could polish off ten beers without thinking. For John, yoga works like replacement therapy for food and drugs.

John's ingenuity is also clear in how he has melded his Catholic faith with his yoga practice. Like many other police officers, John is a faithful gym rat and gets consistent physical release by lifting weights. But the spiritual and emotional benefits of yoga have become essential. In the first couple of years of practice, John's focus was on learning how to balance, staying in the hot room, trying to understand the dialogue, learning to turn down his mind and settle into the breath. With consistent practice, a spiritual aspect of the practice started to emerge. As a regular church-goer, he started to see the yoga dialogue as similar to the priest's homily. He loves the ritual, predictability, and comfort he gets from hearing the same dialogue week after week. Waving his hands around his head while miming the expansion of his brain, John explains to me, "Things open up. Your brain. The room gets fuzzy. I get a sense of enlightenment. I feel like I'm flying, floating in the air." Really concentrating on the homily and the yoga dialogue makes him feel whole.

Five years into his practice, John is really able to "dial in" to a medita-tive focus, a state that stays with him after the practice is over. He describes the state as like the high he felt when he ran a marathon, but more peace-ful. While the damages of war and the brutality he sees on the streets run the risk of dampening his belief in humanity, yoga has strengthened his religious faith. Yoga, in combination with his love for his family, has put him in touch with a spiritual depth the runs deeper than the trauma he has faced.

Witnessing

For survivors, yoga invites awareness of a plane beyond the busy reality of every day, an inner world of acceptance, mystery, and grace. Yogis and meditators have given this awareness many names over the years—the witness, wisdom mind, or original mind.[10] When we access this place of mystery we know we are more than our bodies, more than our individual selves.

When I started reading yogic accounts of this witnessing presence, the first thing I thought of was dissociation—the experience many trauma survivors have had of splitting off from the trauma we were enduring. This is often our first experience of going to a place that cannot be found through the rational mind. The entity that splits off from us watches the trauma from afar, perhaps from the ceiling or the sky. Or the witnessing presence may be lodged in an inanimate object—a wall, a table, a chair, a bedpost, a fence—that holds memory.

Part of the work of healing is to befriend this witness, which is the chronicler of information that the rational mind had to close down to "forget." Bringing the witness into our conscious awareness, and learning what it saw, is both a burden and a gift. The burden is in knowing, forever, the capacity for cruelty in the world. The gift is in knowing our ability to survive what might have seemed to the rational mind, at the time of the original trauma, unsurvivable.

The parallels between the witness as described by yogis and the watching entity that emerges during trauma are fascinating. About the yogic witness, Stephen Cope writes: "There is someone watching the whole thing—the whole storm of thoughts, feelings, and sensations. We're not constantly aware of this, but every now and then we're aware that We, or Some One or Some Thing or Some Alien Force, is watching, witnessing, seeing the whole bloody mess."[11]

This sounds a lot like the split-off observer during trauma—the entity that watches, takes in the whole scene, chronicles the feelings, smells, colors, sounds, and other sensations. Of course, in the yogic tradition the witness is not born of injury, while the observer produced by dissociation is clearly born of trauma. And yet both offer us knowledge of realities beyond the rational.

In the yogic tradition, there is an understanding that the witness operates on a different frequency from left-brain, rational thought processes. "Tuning into this natural mind," yoga teacher Donna Farhi writes, "is rather like tuning into a radio frequency where the broadcast is completely silent and the transmission is felt by the heart rather than heard by the ear."[12] Doesn't that sound like the experience of trauma as well—the experience chronicled in the heart, lodging itself in the deep folds of that precious organ, but not necessarily accessible through one's conscious senses?

The yogic tradition teaches us that with practice, the witness can grow stronger. In trauma theory as well, there is an understanding that working with the patterns and causes of dissociation will make a survivor stronger and build awareness of our gifts, our interconnectedness, our courage.

The connection between the witness born of trauma and the yogic witness is one of the reasons that, when I first became aware of my own yogic witness, it frightened me. It took me back to the witnessing that had been born of deep fear related to losing my father, sexual abuse, and other violence. Once I was able to trace the emotions I was feeling back to the experiences that had given rise to dissociation, I could then experience the yogic witness with less emotional resistance. Over time, I was able to welcome the witness as company, as a presence that can see the bigger picture. Accessing this witness put me in touch with a certain spaciousness, what Pema Chödrön might call the "cool loneliness" that reminds us of our connection to the eternal, to something within us that is wise, kind, nonjudgmental.[13]

Through yoga, it is possible to welcome to consciousness knowledge that might otherwise be cordoned off—including awareness of the experiences that prompted the original dissociation. The more we understand the dynamics of dissociation, the more we understand the yogic witness. And vice versa.

Remembering Your Spirit

In her revelatory book *Soul Talk: The New Spirituality of African American Women,* the poet and professor Akasha Gloria Hull writes that her experience of happiness and self-confidence as an adult is directly related to confronting her early history of sexual and emotional abuse. Her healing led her to see these experiences "less as victimization and more as far-reaching redemption." Survivors who are on a healing path learn how to work it—to recognize the inner resources and special abilities that were first developed as children that can be embellished upon as adults. Hull writes, "Thrown back upon our young selves and our inner resources, when we did not go under, we developed an impressive list of positive assets that include: original thought and creative imagination; independence and self-reliance; awareness of spiritual beings and energies; a sense of a core divine that could not be beaten down or killed."[14]

Hull names spiritual capacities as part of what survivors experience and learn. We come to the mat with these resources, whether named or not. The slow, steady wisdom that comes from regular practice can lead us back to these resources. A willingness to find others who are also searching to reclaim themselves is often part of this journey.

I am reminded of a retreat I participated in at the Furious Flower Poetry Center in Virginia, where a poet and teacher in her fifties spoke about having been locked in a closet when she was a child.[15] Her eyes brimmed with tears as she spoke; this was a woman not used to crying in public and surprised by her own candor. The poet Sonia Sanchez turned to her and said that in "ceremonies" during her meditations she learned to "shake off" memories of being locked in a closet when she was a child. During these rituals she spoke directly to the memory of the woman who had locked her up, saying, "You don't have a hold on me anymore. Leave me now. I am done with you. Leave my body." As Sanchez spoke, the room opened up with awareness, and everybody watched as she demonstrated the shaking she did, with her limbs, her head, her silver hair. A consummate teacher and healer, Sanchez embodied her spiritual practice.

In the 1970s and 1980s there was an expression, "out of the closets and into the streets," that was commonly used by people involved in civil disobedience and other forms of protest to gain civil rights for people across lines of sexuality, race, gender, and class. This is what is happening for people who have been traumatized now, a willingness to manifest our healing, shaking ourselves free, coming out of the closet to each other, healing in community.

In the Secrets, the Stories Are Told

Over the years, one of the characteristics of trauma survivors that has most struck me is how often they do not identify their own courage. This may be because they are so used to coping that they don't have a chance to think about their brave ways. It may be that naming their courage goes against their own sense of humility or quiet determination. It may be because naming what they are up against would feel too disruptive or risky. Whatever the reason, many trauma survivors teach me how gutsy it can be to practice yoga. Not just showing up, but sustaining the practice over the long run.

I think, for example, of a group of people I worked with at the International Women's Partnership for Peace and Justice outside of Chiang Mai, Thailand, who grew up in refugee camps and who are now working there as domestic violence counselors and mental health providers. During our three-day workshop in 2012, this group of activists was totally engaged in their own yoga practice and the intensive workshops. They were willing to talk about how yoga had helped them with their own traumas (sexual violence, the stress involved in growing up as refugees) and were interested in taking yoga back to their communities.

It wasn't until they were debriefing with the two founders of the International Women's Partnership that the activists revealed their bind. While eager to teach yoga, they would need to call it simply "stretching" since the fundamentalist Christian refugees would consider "yoga" blasphemous and dangerous. When I learned about the renaming they will need to do, I was struck by their ingenuity as well as their decision not to tell me about their dilemma. Out of respect for me, perhaps, they had to figure out how to translate what we talked about into acceptable language in the camps.

More than halfway across the world, but actually in my own backyard (in Boston), I saw this quiet courage again, this time in the story of Janelle, a gorgeous, exquisitely fit, forty-year-old Haitian educator who has been practicing yoga and meditation since her twenties. As a woman raised in a tight-knit Seventh-Day Adventist family that attended church several days a week, serendipity is what first brought her to meditation after she happened to see Deepak Chopra on *Oprah*. Finding herself immediately drawn to his conversation about meditation and harmony, Janelle sought out information about meditation on her own, a discovery that led her to take a three-day Transcendental Meditation retreat. As someone who had long questioned many of the doctrines and the exclusivity of the Seventh-Day Adventist theology, she was thrilled by the openness she found at the retreat. To this day, she still remembers floating home after the days spent in meditation, feeling light, happy to be alive. This was the beginning of what has become a lifelong journey that has included a daily yoga and meditation practice, becoming a yoga teacher herself (alongside teaching kickboxing, aerobics, and muscle conditioning), and studying ayurvedic medicine. As she says about herself, "I have a fondness for all things spiritual."

Yoga and meditation have been company for her all these years, including when she secretly terminated a pregnancy after realizing that her partner was not serious about a committed relationship. Yoga also helped her become physically and spiritually stronger after the procedure compromised her immune system. The fact that she couldn't tell her mother or siblings about the procedure or why she was so weak and that they "roll their eyes" when she practices yoga speaks to her own inner strength. When she was healing, she chanted, finding kirtan a form of prayer to send her problems away. When another relationship ended sadly, Janelle's way of dealing with the loss was to focus on a Sanskrit phrase she had learned while studying ayurvedic medicine in Iowa—*sukham dukham anagatam* (which loosely translates to "avert the danger before it happens"). With this mantra she was trying to listen to her still small voice that had said "no" early. This is the guts of an everyday yogi survivor.

I think too about how, after many years of successfully teaching yoga (based on the long-term mentoring from a seasoned yoga teacher), her contract was terminated once new management insisted that she have professional certification. Her devotion to teaching speaks to her own internal compass. She knows another teaching door will open. And she continues to worship regularly with her family at the Seventh-Day

Adventist Church, even as she practices yoga and meditation as well. When I asked Janelle how she handles not talking with her family about the centrality of yoga and meditation in her life, how she copes with being called a "Black blond" or a "space cadet" by family members, she smiled her beautiful smile and said, "I just do more yoga." Meanwhile she passed me her email address, her first name wrapped around the word *vedic,* even her email an act of naming and claiming herself.

Percolating Prana/Ubuntu

> Someone who is searching for clarity always sees more suffering
> than those who do not.
> —T. K. V. Desikachar[16]

Many years ago, a woman I interviewed for a book I was working on described herself as a sponge, absorbing the world's pain wherever she went.[17] Over the years, many yogi trauma survivors I have worked with have resonated with her description. This way of being has its challenges—such simple actions as walking down the street, reading the newspaper, talking with strangers, seeing certain movies can leave people feeling all of the sadness, worry, loss inside of their bodies, absorbing the pain. As the poet Joy Harjo writes, "I've always had a theory that some of us / are born with nerve endings longer than our bodies."[18] When I first identified this about myself, though, I was hesitant to try to change it, thinking that the world could use some of us "extra-sensitive" types, people not willing to walk away from the world's hurts.

It may take a while (okay, maybe decades) to modulate exposure to sadness, grief, and pain. This discipline can include becoming more consciously aware of what we take in and give out to the world. In yoga terms, this is the work of breath control (pranayama), working with our vital energy through the breath, by learning to keep our life force. A sign of sickness or weakness can occur when you allow much of your prana to disperse outside of your body.[19] In my case, learning to be a caretaker while growing up in an alcoholic family and feeling powerless to stop the violence I witnessed resulted in giving away a lot of my prana, which ironically also led me to people with leaky prana as well.

One beauty of yoga is how it teaches you to sense your body not only at the physical level but also at the level of energy. So, part of healing includes sensing when people are dumping prana all over the place and then deciding whether you want to engage or not. Rather than finding ourselves around people whose prana is dispersed (when you then are susceptible to playing the role of the cleanup artist), we can walk in the direction of people who are percolating their own prana—who are sensitive and invested in a just world and also know they need to take care of themselves, regenerate each day.

In his discussion of suffering *(duhkha)*, Desikachar explains that "dust that lands on the skin is harmless, but if only a tiny particle gets into the eye, it is very painful. In other words, someone who is searching for clarity becomes sensitive because the eyes must be open, even if what they see is sometimes very unpleasant. Someone who is searching feels or sees things long before other people do. He or she develops a special insight, a particular kind of sensitivity."[20] This special sensitivity is one of the gifts that may come from injury. But when this sensitivity results in our constant giving away of our life force, we will be drained rather than strengthened in the process.

The ability to see suffering is part of what can make us fully human—what the Nobel Prize–winning spiritual leader of South Africa, Desmond Tutu, has called *ubuntu*.[21] The challenge is to do this while avoiding the pitfalls of exhaustion, feeling overwhelmed and powerless in the process. In *The Heart of Yoga* there are two delightful photos of Desikachar's father, Krishnamacharya, doing extended triangle pose *(utthita trikonasana)* and revolved triangle *(parivrtta trikonasana)*—standing perfectly in balance as he is seeing the world from the front and back with equal clarity and focus.[22] Balancing the prana within us helps to create balance in the world.

To See but Not Dissolve

When working with trauma survivors, a message I try to pass on is about developing an affectionate understanding of the ways we cope. This is the tadasana pose for healing—the absolute foundation. Coping may start with smoking cigarettes and pot while stationed in Afghanistan or bingeing on a neighbor's food when babysitting. It may have been splitting into multiple personalities as a child in the face of too many assaults, or cutting yourself during holiday meals with your biological family. There is a reason that the expression "making a way out of no way" was first used among Black people during slavery—unjust systems compel methods that require extraordinary, often undetectable uses of the imagination.

A huge step in trauma recovery is developing a positive—even humorous—attitude toward our methods of coping and awareness that it could have been worse. We could have killed ourselves (or someone else), overdosed on drugs, or acted out with road rage. Also, the coping methods we adopted often include some creativity—if we can let go of the shame and guilt about them. Trauma survivors tend to be creative. That is often how we first find each other—we connect not through our "dysfunction" but through our ingenuity. Think about it—we uphold the expression "think globally but act locally"—buying, liquor, cigarettes, foods for bingeing, razor blades that support the local economy. We leave all kinds of clues—sometimes so obvious it is amazing it takes people years to figure us out. We try to help others even though we may still be drowning ourselves. And we have macabre, smart-alecky, and idiosyncratic senses of humor.

Developing compassion about how we cope has to be in place before we can understand symptoms and common personality traits that we might want to revise. We need the soft pine needle foundation of compassion before we can start what, in twelve-step programs, they refer to as a "searching and fearless moral inventory" of ourselves. So, read on only if you have the compassion piece down.

- Sometimes trauma survivors think of ourselves as exceptions even when we aren't. Because we lived through extraordinary circumstances, we somehow think we deserve special treatment now even when we don't need it.[23] How this may show up in yoga is thinking we deserve more time with the teacher after class than the others, or thinking we never deserve time with the teacher. Survivors run the risk of living in the land of extremes—all yes, or all no. People may think we were so exceptionally injured that no therapist will be able to help us. Or that no twelve-step program, or group therapy, or yoga program will work. This is why meditation, as a practice of equanimity, may be especially important for survivors. Meditation has a way of reminding us of our precious place in a big universe—we are simultaneously special, and not.

• Trauma survivors sometimes run the risk of taking ourselves too seriously. Maybe because we were told by many people to just "suck it up" or, worse, ignore the trauma all together, we have a hard time letting it go even when we can. Extra sensitive, easily hurt, taking everything personally, afraid everyone is out to get us, somehow, some way, someday. How that plays itself out on the yoga mat is that if someone comes over to adjust us, we might think the sky has fallen and Chicken Little was killed, rather than that the teacher sees that our right hip is competing with the Empire State Building or that the teacher-in-training who is noticing any- and everything that could be "fixed" about our postures is trying too hard herself (i.e. don't take it personally).

• One of the unique survivor qualities is being able to sense that the world is on fire—the earth, our people, are in trouble. We are not the kind to walk down the street and ignore someone who is homeless. We are not the kind to castigate people who talk to themselves, who can't seem to sustain a long-term relationship, who fall into bankruptcy, who can't seem to "get it together." The flip side of this is hypersensitivity—having a hard time living through our days without going on overload, getting totally stressed out, overstimulated. Absorbing the world's pain is both a quality and a liability (since it places us at the center somehow, responsible for responding to, fixing all that is wrong).

The tricky thing about naming these ways of reacting is that much of it is not conscious. Even as I am writing this, I feel like I am telling secrets and putting into words what we have buried with shame. But the behaviors I am talking about are not hustles, not manipulation—they are typically not even conscious enough to be that. The more that trauma survivors see ourselves as part of a community—all of us on paths of healing—the more chance we have to name our reactions and then, when we can, let them go.

This is when practicing balancing poses regularly comes in handy, reminding us not to tip in one direction over the other, or else we will fall. This is when child's pose (balasana) and pigeon (eka pada raja kapotasana) are helpful—poses that encourage humility and a time to take stock. This is where prayer and asanas meet—in that place of humility and gratefulness that can help us reach out but not take on too much. To see but not dissolve. To practice the yoga of karma that is not based on reacting or overreacting. To be watchful, at least at first, reminding ourselves that we are part of communities. We don't have to fix it all ourselves.

Between Fight or Flight

> The inner states [of the autonomic nervous system] resonate with some of the most fundamental of all human emotions—whether individuals feel safe and protected or threatened and endangered. They reflect not only our survival instincts but the mood swings of childhood.
>
> —William J. Broad[24]

Since one symptom for many trauma survivors is our difficulty in getting out of emergency mode, one challenge is to find ways to be less reactive, more balanced in handling what comes our direction. While being stuck in emergency mode partly stems from habit, there is actually a physiological basis for this pattern as well—"how the nervous system helps us defend ourselves."[25] Constantly bracing for the next disaster begins at the level of the sympathetic nervous system that gets caught in what is called "fight or flight" following trauma. Symptoms of fight or flight include a racing heart, tense muscles, and energy surges that are preparing the body to respond to danger. While the fight-or-flight response can literally save people's lives, there is a problem when we get stuck in this mode—always ready to take off, as adrenaline and cortisol (a stress hormone) are constantly "on." The flip side of fight or flight is "freeze or submit," a response by the parasympathetic nervous system, causing us to tremble, shake, feel acid in our stomachs, and feel exhausted. Like fight or flight, freeze or submit is a remarkable way the body responds to danger, by pulling in and closing down in response to danger. But when freeze or submit becomes constant, it can be hard to get out of bed in the mornings or eat a meal without having a nervous stomach.

One of the gifts of healing is beginning to live in a space between fight or flight—feeling neither the need to run all the time or defend ourselves at every turn—and freeze or submit. You could call this space equanimity. For many people, living in this space has to do with timing—knowing what is an emergency and what isn't, refusing to be a drama queen, getting help as soon as possible when there really is something amiss. The space between fight or flight and freeze or submit is one where you can trust that not everything has to be done immediately but also that if something is urgent, you will be able to respond.

Trauma survivors often have trouble with what, in a car, is the timing belt. When working well, that part keeps the pistons firing on time, keeps the car idling but not revved up when standing, allows an automatic transmission to move from first to second to third gear without jerking in the process. Symptoms that more healing might be in order show up when our timing is off—either flat or lethargic when there is a real emergency or revved up, all caffeinated, when calm is needed. I am thinking of an example of a scene between my son, LaMar, and me that occurred only several months after he came to live with me when he was nine. I was washing windows on the first floor when a decades-old storm window came crashing down, shattering glass all over the dining room, including two shards that lodged themselves in my quadriceps. I screamed that kind of guttural scream that you don't necessarily recognize in yourself but lets you know you were caught off-guard. I grabbed paper towels for my leg and a broom to start sweeping when I realized that LaMar had not come downstairs even though the cows in Romania could have heard my scream. When he did come down, he just stood at the door frame with a flat blank face, seeming nonplussed.

You can only imagine what happened next—two trauma survivors meeting at an unlucky pass. I, furious that he didn't come running down to see if I was okay, was clearly triggered by being alone and vulnerable sometimes as a child myself. He was scared out of his mind (revealing expression, huh?) that I was going to blame him for what happened, that I would lash out, or worse, disappear on him. In that moment, I didn't have the level head to see trauma-meeting-trauma, to slow down and hug him, to assure him everything would be okay. Instead, I started to yell at him—"Why didn't you come down right away? Don't you know how to show concern for someone you love?"—singularly hurtful on my part. I cringe at how poorly I handled the situation, my trauma-based response still seared in my brain.

I give this example because trauma can throw our timing off. And if there are two trauma survivors involved—both having misfired timing belts—you have the potential for hurt feelings, fears that don't get named, accusations that stick when hugs and softness and slowing down are in order. This is what yoga can do—start to protect us from the impact of collision while teaching us a sense of timing. Yoga has the ability to calm the autonomic nervous system (by creating a balance between its two parts—the sympathetic and parasympathetic nervous system) while teaching us that pause in between the postures can be practiced in conversations, and in crises as well. Now is not the time, for example, to yell at your son. Hugging would be better. So many lessons. No time like the present to start again.

Willing to Be Schooled

> We are not supposed to live this life pain-free. That is not honest.
> Addiction to prescription drugs is a way to avoid pain when what
> I needed to do was look at it straight in the face. Self-medication
> closes people up, isolates people, makes people become selfish.
> Choosing another way is a way of living fully.
> —Chris Gibbs

A key characteristic that stands out for me about yogi survivors is their guts. Guts in getting out of tight spots. Guts in finding the type of yoga that works for them. Guts in taking a break from yoga if it feels like too much. Guts in creating healing communities. Among those I have known over the years, my friend Chris Gibbs offers one of the most compelling stories of why guts is a four-letter word—both in the trouble he has found himself in and the guts he has shown to get out of it.

Chris is a thirty-two year-old man of Italian and Mohawk descent who grew up on Cape Cod. He has been adventurous since he was a young child. His father tells a story of finding Chris climbing up their porch when he was two years old, shinning up ropes, ladders, and other high places. This risk-taking followed him into adulthood as he became a certified skydiver, cliff jumper, and motorcyclist. As he tells me, "I basically played hard. I spent a lot of time wrecking my body." His on-the-edge living resulted in two accidents—one when he was boating with friends. He was goofing around in the water with three young women when the driver of the boat accidentally hit the women, killing one of them. Chris was there when this happened, saying it was the most gruesome scene he had ever witnessed, with blood everywhere. He dove down under the water as deep and as long as he could, to no avail. He had night terrors for years after that, haunted by what he might have done differently, how he might have averted her violent death. The doctors he sought prescribed pain medication that did nothing to ease the PTSD symptoms and everything to walk him into an addiction to prescription drugs.

A few years later he faced another accident, this time while on his motorcycle. He was taking a tricky mountain turn when the bike crossed over the yellow line and then went under him. He was thrown back into a cow fence, his back wrapping around it like a C curve. Although he somehow managed to not break his back, his rotator cuff was severed, his feet badly injured, and his patella cut in half. The doctors prescribed morphine and Percocet. Each time he returned in pain, the doctor wrote another prescription. Chris became addicted to the medicine again as his world seemed to get smaller and smaller. Between the emotional fallout from the boating accident and the motorcycle crash, Chris spent two years on heavy pain medication, with little success.

When he first found his way to a yoga class, he had no idea that it was an advanced class. As was his nature, he threw himself right in, only to injure himself again. This understandably left him skeptical about yoga until a year later when a roommate convinced him to try a Bikram class since it is designed especially for people healing from injuries. He immediately knew that he and yoga were a match. He felt one hundred percent in tune with the words, the energy, and the heat, his whole body in harmony, like nothing he had ever experienced. Following the class he asked the teacher what he needed to do to become an instructor. She shook her head, nonplussed, and said he could start by taking a second class. Within a month, Chris was seeing dramatic healing. Without surgery he regained full range of motion in his rotator cuff. He was sleeping better since the night terrors were substantially diminished and his balance improved. In addition, he was able to walk in an upright and easy way after years of creaking around from his many daredevil adventures.

As he has deepened his practice, more of the tools have been revealed to him, including clarity of mind, increased discipline, voluminous energy, and a "willingness to be schooled." For Chris one of the biggest benefits of his practice is the humility it nurtures, a quality that he associates with needing to look oneself in the mirror. He tells me, "you have to face yourself. Give up ego, give up pride. You have to get past the notion that yoga is not for guys, to get to a point where you know that yoga is for everybody." And, he says, "You need to be willing to look pain straight in the face, to look at the cobwebs, the memories, what haunts us." For Chris this has meant looking deeply at the boat accident involving his friend, coming to accept that it happened and that he couldn't save her. And, he tells me, "It has meant asking myself why I beat up my body so much, why I needed to live on the edge to feel like I was living at all."

Chris's life also gives an example of how traits that sometimes lead people to injury are often ones they can claim in a new way through yoga. The adventurous spirit that led Chris initially to push his body too hard is what led to the addiction to prescription drugs. Yoga has enabled him to transform that spirit into discipline and enthusiasm for the practice. It has brought him clarity of mind that, when he speaks about it, can move him to tears. It took guts for him to refuse to stay hooked on painkillers. It was brave for him to recognize that his risk-taking could cost him his life. He realized that his sense of adventure needed to be more internal, at the level of spiritual questing rather than conquering a road or jumping from cliffs. For Chris, pushing himself comes easily. Slowing down, taking stock, and easing into postures is harder.

Of course finding a middle ground is a process. On any given day, Chris is likely to teach an intensive yoga class in the morning, do construction work all day, and then go back to the studio again on his way home. He says he can't stop his enthusiasm. The ancient energy embodied in the poses and the determination on people's faces as they practice keep him pumped up to do as much yoga as his body will allow. It is true, he reminds me, that the chances of getting injured are a whole lot less in a supervised yoga studio than they were when he was jumping out of planes and off of cliffs. But he can't help but be a survivor.

Bat Consciousness

The world throws back a language, the empty space rising between hills speaks an open secret then lets the bats pass through, here or there, in the dark air.
—Linda Hogan[26]

In yoga, a multitude of poses are named after birds and animals—crow, eagle, bird of paradise, cow face pose, cobra, rabbit, just to name a few. There is no pose named after the bat, which is unfortunate given how bats have abilities that closely resemble the characteristics of trauma survivors. In a gorgeous essay by Linda Hogan, the Native American environmentalist and poet writes about discovering two bats that had been grounded in grass after a dramatic fall in temperature stopped them in mid-flight. She watched them try to recuperate, which primarily involved mating for three days, until finally, the male, exhausted and depleted, died as the female flew away, a new body inside her.

In the process of witnessing, Hogan began to discover that it is "the world-place bats occupy that allows them to be of help to people, not just because they live inside the passageways between earth and sunlight, but because they live in double worlds of many kinds."[27] Like bats, survivors often live outside and inside of our bodies simultaneously, traversing the boundary of skin without a sound as warning. We are often most sensitive to dusk and dawn, the most energetically alive times of day and night, shape-shifting our way through transitions.

Like bats, survivors can be highly intuitive. Part of hypervigilance is being intuitive—learning how to pick up on what people say in words as well as what they are saying with their body language, anticipating danger before it comes, talking in ways to elicit truths that might otherwise not emerge, doubling back on conversations to cross-check reality. Like bats, we have learned to get messages from uncanny places, willing to consider all kinds of evidence to help piece together a livable space, a coherent story. Bats are able to get vital messages from the architecture of buildings, a wind channel, a church steeple, a long corridor of energy at the end of a one-way street. Hogan writes that for the bat, "everything answers, the corner of a house, the shaking of leaves on a wind-blown tree, the solid voice of bricks."[28] Survivors also have had to find our way through unnamed territory, moments that had no words—that were buried in secrets. Survivors often live in empty spaces, sometimes afraid to leave our own houses, sometimes afraid to return.

Some of what people seek in yoga is a way to recognize and consolidate knowledge that we have had but have not necessarily understood. Like bats we "hear the sounds that exist at the edges of our lives."[29] This is what yoga allows. Over time, it is as if long forgotten channels of knowledge open up, messages we have gathered from many directions, some in words, some in music, from the smell of a grandmother's room, a child's baby food, the colors of autumn. For bats, "even noisy silences speak out in a dark dimension of sound that is undetected by our limited hearing in the loud, vibrant land in which we live."[30] Practicing yoga, getting quiet in meditation, and breathing deeply allows us to hear silences in new ways, to detect messages that we could not make sense out of before.

Hogan notes that a bat hears "a world alive in its whispering songs."[31] That is what can happen in yoga, too. Feeling the world alive in new ways, feeling ourselves to be a part of the ocean, the wind, the trees. The sage sociologist Maurie Schwartz said that he used to be afraid of death until he realized that instead of being a drop of water alone in a huge ocean, he began to see himself as a wave, a part of the ocean like light is to sky. Bats may already know themselves to be part of a larger design. Yoga helps teach us about this.

For survivors, getting out into the world some days can feel daunting, finding your way to a new studio, teacher, classmates, and postures. The bat intuition that some humans possess is the sense that there is healing out there even when there are no obvious signs along the way, or they are elusive, ineffable, not yet well marked.

"Can't Keep Living in a Teacup"

Trauma often robs people of a sense that an experience has not just a beginning but an ending, too. Some part of us remains frozen in a destructive experience that is ceaselessly reenacted, never coming to a conclusion. This is one reason that many survivors appreciate yoga teachers who count down the seconds, from beginning to end, of the individual yoga poses. The counting lets us know that the experience of the pose is finite, and therefore enables us to go into it with all of our selves instead of hanging back.

One of the benefits of getting unfrozen (in our feelings, actions, plans, responses to people) is how it allows us to get on with our lives—to live as big a life as we would like. My friend Anna Dunwell, owner of the yoga studio Soul Sanctuary, sometimes tells me, "We can't keep living in a teacup all of our lives." Anna keeps stepping into the center of her own life, to the center of her life's work (dharma). Over the years she has been endlessly inventive at rising to life's challenges, incorporating her artistic background in textiles and design into the creation of a gorgeous yoga studio; setting up intricate round-the-clock care for her mother so that she can live out her final years with Anna and her family rather than going to a nursing home; implementing a cutting-edge yoga curriculum for her work with torture survivors.

Many of us find ourselves hanging out at the periphery of life until we get the support we need to step into the center. We live at the margins in our work, our relationships, our creativity, our bodies, and our spiritual development. This attachment to the sidelines is often based in fear. If I step into the center, will I be enough? Will I get the support I need to stay there? And even with help from people who love me, do I have what it takes to let all of my creative abilities develop?

Stepping into the center of our lives is a way to feel fully alive. The Yoga Sutras say that direct experience, whenever possible, is superior to that which is lived through others. Nurturing our own gifts is better than living through other's accomplishments. It is the difference between watching the TV show *Dancing with the Stars* and dancing yourself, the difference between traveling to Ghana and seeing the photos of someone else's trip.

Learning to live a life rather than watch it happen is one of the promises of the asanas as well as focused concentration (dharana) and meditation (dhyana). These practices put us into mindful states of being that can bring us the clarity we need to make it to the center—of ourselves, and our lives.

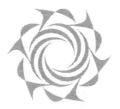

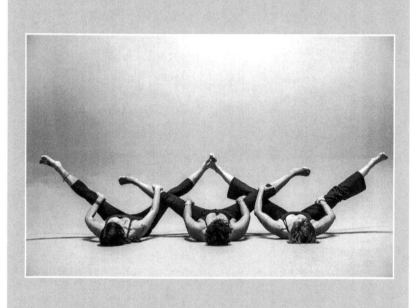

PART III

Hide
and
Seek

The Circuitous
Path of Healing

One of the lessons that yoga teaches is how elusive, time consuming, and unpredictable healing can be. Many of the processes of becoming whole take place behind the scenes, over long stretches of time and invisible to the casual observer. The healing processes are never exactly the same for any two people, and cannot be reduced to generic recipes but have to be adapted for different circumstances.

Healing is also circuitous, erratic. If we are practicing yoga for healing purposes, we may see progress not only in our poses, but also in our relationships, our stamina, and our ability to stay centered even as the world spins. But we may then go through a period when we have difficulty communicating with anybody, when just getting to the yoga studio is all we can do—if that—and savasana the only pose we are interested in practicing.

This unpredictability is what causes many yogis to recommend that we cultivate contentment (*santosa,* the second niyama). Such contentment, such equanimity, can often be found by simply slowing down, moving through space on the mat and off as if it were warm honey, not slippery ice. Thus many trauma survivors on a healing path find themselves paying close attention to the daily rituals in their lives, including what they eat and drink, seeing eating as a spiritual practice that three times a day allows them to become exquisitely conscious of their movements, feelings, thoughts. This is no small event for survivors, being willing to consciously pay attention at the level of sensations—choosing not to throw food down our throats to stifle feelings of anger, loneliness, and fear, but to sit with those feelings. Such a practice helps people start to distinguish between savoring and craving, between spiritual hunger and hunger for food, between eating to live and living to eat. Such a practice means being willing to move beyond habit and familiarity, to stay attuned to, rather than numb to, what comes our direction.

The hide-and-seek nature of healing means recognizing that it is easier to stay steady during some yoga practices than others. Some days you can pop right into bow pose *(dhanurasana),* other days, not. Sometimes you stay cool when your teen daughter comes home two hours late, while at other times you yell, finding yourself apologizing later. Learning to stay in a pose, even when the sensations are difficult, comes from practicing contentment. This is a state of mind that can help people weather the ups and downs of healing.

When I am honest, the peaceful patience that I find on the mat is often the exception, not the rule, in my everyday life. Hide-and-seek not only relates to the uneven process of understanding and healing the body. It also characterizes the process of practicing the principles of yoga off the mat. It is a process we see, and then don't; yearn for, and then forget; practice, and then practice some more. These lessons can come from uncanny places: while riding a bike home from a practice as I chronicle in the story "Sanskrit on the Bike" or while watching a squirrel build a new nest as described in "Black Walnuts and a Hurricane." Healing from trauma can feel like being willing to walk in and out of a tornado, each time seeking the eye of the storm. Practicing yoga can be like finding safety in that place until the weather passes.

Sanskrit on the Bike

I am just back from a yoga retreat in which I had an inspired time—the result of a combination of exquisite teaching; a gorgeous lake that I could see from my window; time with Diane, my closest of kin; and wonderful wasabi tofu and sesame kale. I drove home through Sunday-night traffic feeling more like I was flying than strapped into a slow-moving car, arriving home to my marvelous daughter and a burst of energy that helped me write late into the night.

When I woke the next morning, I was excited to go to my yoga class, eager to find the new space in my hips and shoulders that I had experienced during the retreat. Only my practice didn't go as planned. First, although my body made it to the studio, I am not sure my breath ever made it through the door. During practice I felt as though I could barely inflate my lungs. My sacrum felt tender and I was having difficulty listening to the teacher. I couldn't get myself to care about the practice. Several times I had to talk myself out of just slipping quietly out of the room. Hearing the teacher caution the class against skipping poses, I realized that she was speaking to me—as I was the only one in the room not doing the pose—clearly trying to motivate me out of one long corpse pose (savasana) and back into the practice. I wasn't tired. I was just uninspired, foggy, disconnected.

I spent most of the bike ride home listening to my internal voices: "Why do you bother to save your money to go on an annual retreat if you return in worse shape than when you went? Maybe yoga isn't working for you anymore. There were some poses that you couldn't do well today but that you could do ten years ago. What's happening?"

The voices kept at it. Who even knows why these voices were screaming, but they were. The aftermath of trauma seems to have a decibel and timing that is all its own, with "I am not enough" and "I can't do it right" its central refrain.

Fortunately, it finally dawned on me that the lessons I could practice from my yoga retreat weren't going to happen on the mat that day. In fact, it was on the bike that I was practicing yoga . . . moving my way through reciting some of the first two limbs of yoga, the laws of life (yamas) and rules of living (niyamas), focusing on the ones that seemed most relevant to me at that moment—starting with nonviolence (*ahimsa*—which I needed to practice toward myself). After ahimsa I added non-attachment *(aparigraha)*, to remind myself not to become invested in the outcome of yoga, to let the practice evolve. Then I added simplicity *(sauca)* in hopes that I could calm my scattered mind. And then contentment (santosa)— being satisfied with riding my bike on a pretty morning. And finally, I arrived at devotion *(ishvara-pranidhana)*, the loving spirit that links people to the earth and beyond.[1]

When I finished practicing, I realized that the biggest lesson from the weekend had almost nothing to do with the actual poses, the physical practice, and everything to do with working the spiritual limbs, starting with turning those critical, exacting voices around to a kinder place.

But soon the critical voices started again, until I caught myself. "Go through the wheel again, Becky," I told myself—nonviolence, nonattachment, simplicity, contentment, devotion. "Say them in Sanskrit, too. Use them as a mantra if you have to. Practice this on the bike. One turn of the pedals, one word, one turn, one word. See if you can arrive home safely, inside the sounds of the Sanskrit words." Which I did.

Black Walnuts and a Hurricane

After years of making a nest in the eaves of my roof, which I finally blocked last winter, my local squirrel is building a nest in the tree just outside my study window. I marvel at the hope and audacity of such a move since, not even a week ago, this region was hit by a hurricane that was so powerful that between my immediate neighbors and me, we lost five trees, some of which had been standing for well over half a century. The squirrel lost her nest as well. The biggest and oldest of the remaining trees is the one where this squirrel is now building her new nest.

I marvel at all the work the squirrel puts into the project—removing whole branches from lower limbs and then carrying them up to the nest, poking and prodding to find a place to tuck in further reinforcements. With this front row seat, I realize that I will be able to watch this squirrel for the months to come, to see what becomes of this nest that, within just a few short days, has become as big as the top shelf of my refrigerator.

I tell you about this squirrel because her activity reminds me of what transpires during the ups and downs of healing. First, there is the injury, which for her came in the form of a storm—unexpected, unpredictable, destructive. For us, as for her, the injury then necessitates building a new nest. Maybe it will be in an old tree, maybe in a new one, but wherever it is, it must be a securely built place of refuge, perched in a position of safety. To create this haven we too must run around like squirrels, look- ing hard for all the materials we need—a skilled therapist, a yoga studio with sensitive teachers, books on trauma and healing, friends who really understand. If the nest has to be built high up in the tree, hard to get to, we may need a lot of time. We may have to go to workshops, trainings, conferences, and other gatherings of like-minded people who are also trying to figure out how to rebuild their nests. This may require us to take time off from our jobs, or even find a more flexible, less toxic one.

As we rebuild the nest we must ask ourselves what will ensure that it will keep us safe if there is another storm, cold winds, rainy days, snow on the branches. What reinforcements might I need now that I didn't have before? Am I making this rebuilding harder than it needs to be? Am I putting too much energy into a relationship or a job that is draining me, without it giving me enough to replenish the reserves I am spending? Am I burdening myself with fear that if I leave the nest for one quick minute, the whole thing will disappear? Can I let go of some of that worry?

The effort of rebuilding may be why the squirrel outside my window seems to stop after every few foraging trips, taking time to crack open another black walnut, clearly scheduling regular rest and rejuvenation periods into her labors. Makes me wonder if I have given myself the rest and nourishment I need to make my nest strong enough to last through the seasons. I have been noticing that this particular squirrel has been working alone the last few days, doing all of that hauling and chewing and redecorating on her own. I don't know if that's the norm for squirrels, but I do know that if I were doing all the work by myself, I'd be one lonely squirrel. In my own journey to healing, I knew I had to find a yoga studio to be with others, to take time to talk with friends, to avail myself of all kinds of help, in order to find the most direct route to making my new nest. And once I had my nest, I figured out ways to snuggle in at night, safe and warm, below the wind's channel.

Squirrel wisdom: work hard on your nest but not so hard that you exhaust yourself before you are finished; make it secure, but not so far up in the tree that you won't ever have any company in your nest; always keep on hand a stash of black walnuts that you can munch on when a little fortification is in order; take time between your labors to renew yourself. And know that no matter how bad the storm that destroyed your previous nest, you can rebuild—and keep rebuilding, as necessary.

Inspecting the Body

My friend Adrienne, a talented modern choreographer and dancer, talks about the practice of yoga as one where she lifts her body up, as they do at the mechanics on a hydraulic lift, in order to inspect it—as she says to herself, "How is that right hip that was replaced four years ago doing today?" Then she inspects the one replaced a year ago, seeing that the second is making an even more remarkable recovery than the first. Six weeks postsurgery and Adrienne is already inspecting her body with bow pose, standing head-to-knee, locust, and rabbit. She asks herself, "How are those arms and legs, still limber and fierce from years of jumps and turns?" Six weeks after surgery and Adrienne is hoisting her strong dancer's body up for inspection.

This "inspection of the body from down under" approach teaches me how change is the one common denominator in practice. For a long time I was under the impression that once we find our bodies—in the multiple, often unpredictable ways that we do that—we can keep them, only to realize that our awareness of our body parts can come and go. This makes sense since the body is completely reconstituted at the molecular level throughout our lives. But it has taken me a long time to see that getting to know the body is similar to how workers paint the Golden Gate Bridge in San Francisco. The crew painstakingly starts at one end, painting the spanning cables, the side cables, the top and the bottom of the bridge, one section at a time until they reach the other end. Then they start over again. They are never not painting. The bridge is always in process.

I am reminded of a story the Buddhist and Quaker writer Mary Rose O'Reilley tells in her hilarious and brave memoir, *The Barn at the End of the World*, about her stays at Thich Nhat Hanh's Plum Village in France.[2] During one of her extended stays she was told to sort through twigs and branches for her work shift, neatly putting them in piles according to size. Then, the next shift she was told to mess up the piles, spread the twigs and branches out over the soft ground. The next day, O'Reilley was instructed to start her organizing again. A lesson in total futility, for sure. But also one about mindfulness—being mindful in whatever we are doing even if we start again the next day in exactly the same place. This is much of what we do in life, really—start with the dishes again, start with being patient with our children again, start with stretching into child's pose (balasana) again. The body appears to be like that as well, teaching us about mindfulness—and listening. For trauma survivors, this may be even more challenging.

Understanding the body as a process rather than static means that even though I now live inside of my body most of the time, there are still parts of my body that play hide-and-seek with me. This is when the body is talking. I am reminded of how, fifteen years ago, the woman I had been in a long-term, lively, and enchanting relationship with left—much to my surprise. In the following months, as I grieved, whole strips of my skin peeled off—from my face, my hands, my feet. At the time I was dumbfounded by this molting. I had never seen anything like it. Nor had my friends or my trusty health care professional. Retrospectively, though, this "symptom" made sense. The biggest organ in my body, my skin, and the one most visible to the world, was announcing that this big interracial relationship was ending. And that there were aspects of the relationship I had outgrown. My skin was peeling off, a living, breathing example of needing to stretch in new ways.

I think, too, about how there was a period recently when I felt as if part of my abdomen was missing, that I couldn't find myself there. (This is how I used to feel about my whole body.) I didn't know what to make of this until I realized that, since my period stopped coming a year ago, something big *was* missing. When this ordinary, spectacular cycle in my fallopian tubes, ovaries, and uterus stopped, some fundamental, affirming process was no longer happening. This is why I spent months feeling a void, as if part of my abdomen was gone.[3]

There are lessons we can learn from these sometimes funny, typically unnamed bodily symptoms. Yoga provides a space and place to do this—to make sense out of our body's changes. Looking back, I understand why, during the seasons when I couldn't sense my abdomen, I would wake up in the morning craving Breath of Fire (*kapalabhati*, forty to sixty rapid exhalations through the nose while pulling the belly button to the spine). Then I would practice a few *nauli* rolls (using breath to suck in and then rotate the abdominal muscles laterally). Both were ways I found to massage my abdominal organs in order to wake up part of my body again. It makes sense that for years I raised my arm toward the sky in my sleep often, unconsciously lifting up memories stuck in my shoulder and neck. It makes sense that my wise friend continues to put her body up on the yoga lift, inspecting her body's changes so she can continue to create thrilling choreography. The body sometimes brings us realizations before our minds do.

The Devil and the Muse

In yoga philosophy, one way that the "two steps forward and one step back" nature of healing is explained is with the concept of *samskaras*. Samskaras are old patterns that are etched into our consciousness, ruts in our thinking and feeling that we can easily fall back into until we create new patterns of thought and action. Yoga philosopher Steven Cope describes samskaras as "little tracks, little vectors, little ruts in the muddy road. The next time a car travels that road, these muddy ruts will have hardened into permanent fixtures, and the car wheels will want to slide into them. Indeed, it's easier to steer right into them than to try to avoid them."[4]

The process of breaking old samskaras isn't an easy one, most obviously for survivors since trauma has its way of leaving deep tracks of repressed memory in our consciousness. The challenges of breaking old samskaras is poignantly articulated by Tia, an intensive care nurse and longtime yogi whom I met when we were participating in a teacher training in Bali. Her healing has been one of hide-and-seek, courage, and tenacity.

Tia grew up in France, working for many years in an intensive care unit at a major hospital in Paris, caring for people with HIV, those in septic shock after surgery, the sickest of the sick. Among those she worked with was a woman who was having a severe episode of symptoms related to lupus, an autoimmune disease. Tia cared for her for four months, saying that she and her other patients taught her what it means to "save my heart." She found herself asking, "Who is waking who up? I am there to wake them up, but really, they are waking me."

Several years later, Tia was diagnosed with lupus, a disease that was by then too familiar to her, the limits of Western medicine for treating it clear to her as well. The combination of having left a high-stress job, losing a lover to cancer, needing to separate herself from her family, and facing her own diagnosis propelled her on a quest to seek healing outside of the Western model. Her multiyear trek to explore yoga and Buddhism took her to India, Tibet, Vietnam, Thailand, and Bali, where she did lengthy pilgrimages, purifications, and intensive yoga, including a practice of poses specifically designed for healing lupus.[5]

Her increasing devotion to yoga helped keep the lupus at bay. When she left France for Asia, she had lesions on her face and body. Those lesions cleared up almost completely. Almost all of the other major symptoms of the disease, including pain, exhaustion, internal lesions, general weakness, and susceptibility to illness either left her or never manifested. Her energy level and stamina increased. Despite this progress, she still sabotaged herself by smoking and doing drugs that she knows compromise her immune system. Several years into practicing yoga and meditation, she still turns to cigarettes and other drugs for company and to numb difficult feelings.

For Tia, this contradiction partly stems from not knowing how to deal with her life force, what she describes as her light. She explains, "so many times I have sought the light in my life—to find the big light that is in my heart. And to feel the big light in my heart, but then to realize the terror, the absolute panic I feel when I see that light because, in my mind, shining that light in a big way is dangerous—such a light will invite violence, damage." This light is her muse and creativity that make her feel abundantly alive and afraid of her own consciousness. Faced with that contradiction, she turns to drugs. And sometimes she leaves her body, a strategy that the lead teacher in the training called her attention to several times. Because the teacher had her own trauma history, Tia trusted her to help—to stare down her fears by breathing into parts of her body that had been closed down. As she said, "I have been working for many years to do this work now. I couldn't find the key to open this door before."

Her honesty about her addictions is brave partly because the deeper someone goes on a spiritual path, the harder it can be to be upfront about the contradictions they are grappling with. What she describes as the roller coaster of her healing stems from trying to heal emotionally, physically, and spiritually at the same time. If she puts one aspect on hold to deal with another, then she falls out of balance. Meanwhile, she knows that if she puts off her yoga practice, her joints will begin to hurt and she will have lupus symptoms that, when her practice is consistent, are minimal.

Her story is also brave since childhood trauma was exacerbated by adult traumas—including secondary trauma from hospital work. Getting out from underneath the traumas has taken years. She is not alone among fellow travelers who have impressive experience with long-term meditation, yoga, and pilgrimages but who still struggle with addictions. Her courage is in telling complicated truths, that her addictions escalated during a stressful lengthy visit to see her family in France and then subsided again once she left. That she still smoked despite having signed a contract in a yoga certification program that she would consume no drugs or alcohol during her training. The devil (her addictions) and the muse (her quest) are sidling up to each other, her tenacity promising to let compassion win out, truthfulness guide her. As she told me, "healing has come to me drop by drop, not like a shower."

Beginning with Tadasana

Yoga is like the ocean. It goes up and down. You have these days
when you are strong, you can stay in a posture for a long time.
Then there are days when you crumble immediately. There are days
when my knees don't bother me at all. Then there are days when I
can barely stand up. There is no doubt that this yoga is constantly
changing.

—John Brown[6]

Fluctuations in healing are one reason why yogis emphasize cultivating contentment (santosa)—a willingness to ride the ups and downs,
in practice and in life. Such contentment asks us to distinguish between
desires, particularly desires that fuel discontent and yearning. In her book
Compassion, Buddhist writer Christina Feldman offers a generous and
helpful discussion about desire.[7] Feldman clarifies that there are four
kinds of desire, three of which are not the causes of suffering. These are
desires that humans can, in fact, nurture. The first desire is for self-care,
an elemental need (wanting to brush your teeth, eat healthy food). They
are desires that don't leave a "mental residue" and are "answerable." The
second is wholesome longings, the longing for connectedness, freedom,
and peace. These are longings for revolution, liberation struggles that can
inspire and motivate us. They give life shape and direction and remind
us that the seeds of freedom live within us. The third desire is spiritual
urgency—the desire to help, heal, find refuge, sincerity, and compassion.
This desire awakens humans. All three of these desires are answerable.

It is only the fourth desire—craving—that can bring suffering. It has
no end. It is an unquenchable thirst. Craving takes the experience of
savoring something and exaggerates it. This craving can include lusting
after star-studded love, Rolex watches, or the perfect château in Paris. It
can look like striving for a perfect posture, wishing your body (job, life,
relationship) looked like someone else's, wanting to be somewhere else.

A recent example of the distinction between savoring and craving in
my own life occurred when a friend came over with an entire meal of

delectable treats—grilled vegetables and the makings for butternut and ginger soup, salad with barley and *edamame,* cherries, and dark chocolate. I was ravenous, having run through my day without eating enough. Deciding I would be more patient with the preparation for the meal if I ate a little before, my friend sat me down with a portobello mushroom she had grilled with vinegar, oil, and lime, still hot from the hickory coals. Knowing I would only have one mushroom in anticipation of the whole meal later, I slowly savored each of the four bites. At that moment, I am not sure anything had ever tasted better, literal groans of pleasure came out as my eyes rolled back in a food-drunken way. Time seemed to spread out, opening up across the kitchen table. Savoring took its sweet time. It was in no rush, adoring rather than consuming the pleasure.

Later that evening, when we sat down to eat together, no bite was as delicious, delectable, or timeless as the first taste of portobello, as I found myself chasing the experience I had with the appetizer again, wanting it to be the same. My experience had shifted from simply knowing the object to wanting to possess it, have it, make it happen. It shifted from going deep into the experience to skimming the surface. As Stephen Cope explains, "Yogis saw that human beings wish to devour, to possess, to have objects of pleasure—people, places, and things. They saw, too, that objects cannot really be possessed. However, objects *can* be known. And it turns out that it is *knowing* the object that creates the happiness."[8]

Craving causes suffering when it leads to a sense of insufficiency and a diminished sense of inner completeness. Craving has an element of assuming that joy lives outside of ourselves. Craving also easily gets us caught up in trying to prove ourselves, constantly fearful of judgment. Many trauma survivors struggle with a sense of inadequacy—that we don't do our practice well enough, that we don't know enough, try hard enough. And sometimes people feel bad about having any desires at all. That fear can include having trouble asking for big or little things, being afraid that if you take anything, you will somehow owe somebody. Or, if you get what you desire and then lose it, you will have to go through missing it again. Better to just not want it to begin with.

It is okay to attach to a desire to be seen as deserving and worthy. It is more than okay to desire peace and justice. It is more than okay to seek refuge, guidance. I keep thinking about the tadasana pose, the standing pose where it all begins. Trees start from a place of sturdy desire—for earth, water, wind, safety. Trees don't take more water, earth, shelter than they need. They don't crave more than they need. Be a tree with your desires. Start from the earth and build upward.

Three Goats and Two Hens

The sacred is always simple.
—Hugh Milne[9]

The circuitous nature of healing is partly why long-term yogis say to keep it simple. All the elaborations that develop with practice—the latest attire, fancy retreats, state-of-the-art studios, the turning-ourselves-inside-out postures—can distract us from simply getting to the mat.

This link between simplicity (sauca) and contentment (santosa) reminds me of a parable I heard from a rabbi many years ago. There was this family that lived in a small house—a mother and father, two children, a dog and two cats. They went to the rabbi and said, "Rabbi, our house is so small, too small. What ever shall we do?" The rabbi said, "I know exactly how to cure this problem. Go out and ask the big family who lives around the corner to live with you." The people say to the rabbi, "Are you sure?" and he replies, "Yes, I'm sure." The family invites the extended family to come live with them, trying their best, still feeling crowded. The next month they return to the rabbi, "Rabbi, rabbi, our house is too small, what ever shall we do?" The rabbi says, "I have the perfect solution. Ask the three goats and two hens that reside in the barn down the way to join you. This will answer your problems." The people shake their heads, still dutiful to the rabbi, making the trek to invite the goats and hens to their house.

A month later, filled past the gills, they return to the rabbi. "Rabbi, rabbi, what ever shall we do? Our house is too small." The rabbi says, "I know what to do. Ask the traveling salesman to join your house. That will solve it." The family travels back, shaking their heads, opening their doors to the salesman when he comes by with his wares. A month passes, the family distraught, now living with the family from down the street, three goats and two hens, and the traveling salesman. They return to the rabbi saying, "Rabbi, rabbi, what shall we do? Our house is too small." The rabbi looks up and says, "Tell the family, the three goats, two hens, and the traveling salesman that the time has come for them to leave. Then see how it feels. See if the problem you first came with is still with you once they are gone."

You see, three goats, and two hens, an extended family from down the street, and the traveling salesman are too much. What you had before all that might have been just enough. The sacred might more often move into your small house if there is a stool to sit on, a corner to care for, a kettle to fill with the finest chai. The sacred is allergic to clutter. The sacred lives in the simplest of poses, the quietest of practices, the feel of the morning as the stars duck into their sky.

The Possibility of "Eventually"

> The practice of yoga will be firmly rooted when it is maintained
> consistently and with dedication over a long period.
> —Patanjali[10]

One of the lucky characteristics of yoga is how it gives immediate relief.
Sometimes people can notice distinct differences in how they feel within
just a few classes. One woman I began working with, who had survived
the genocide in Zimbabwe even as many family members perished, hadn't
been able to sleep through the night for years. Her restlessness made her
hesitant to travel, to stay at friends' houses, afraid to wake people up from
their sleep. After her first day she slept like a baby, stunned that such a
thing was possible. She came to class the next morning beaming—not
only because she was rested, but also because of the possibility for travel
and visits that such sleeping might allow.

A young woman I work with came bounding into her second class
thrilled because doing yoga was the first time she felt like she was dancing
since injury had forced her to give up her life as a modern jazz dancer. The
music playlist and the flowing sequence made her feel light on her feet and
helped her find a sensual rhythm in her body again. A transgender activist I
worked with in Thailand said that from the first time she did yoga, she felt
she had found something that made room for her spirit, as the dialogue
encouraged her to come fully into her body. A vet I worked with reported
that the intensity of the practice kept his anxiety at bay, breathing something he was willing to try on for size as long as he could keep moving.

It is lucky that many benefits from yoga are obvious. They help when,
as the days and then weeks of doing yoga increase, skepticism and resistance might start to arise. There are many reasons why it is hard to keep
doing yoga, to come to class even when you feel like ditching. This reality
may be one reason why yoga philosopher Patanjali emphasizes consistency in one of the first of the 196 aphorisms for yoga.[11] When I think
about the master teachers and yogis I have known, they tend to live predictable lives. They go to bed early and get up early. They eat healthy food,

lots of fruits and vegetables, and are careful about not eating too much. They practice every day. They avoid places where there is over-the-top artificial stimulation—television, malls, violent movies, drunkenness, lots of yelling. As longtime contemplative practitioner Geri Larkin writes, "Quiet surrounds them. They move with grace and with humor. Even when there is a crisis, there is always a calmness about them which reaches past the crisis into a sky of wisdom, where they choose their reaction to the situation."[12]

This is the rub. Consistency and predictability can be especially hard for people who have seen trauma. It can feel boring for people who grew up trying to manage other people's crises. Yoga may feel tedious to vets who awaited the next operation or the chaos of people screaming in pain. Predictability can feel like something is missing, an eerie quiet before a storm for people who have been around gunshots and watched people die in front of them. For many survivors, having a sense of routine can itself be scary. Consistency and dedication also seem to run counter to the human predilection toward newness and invention. I am remembering a yoga student who is also a surgeon who confessed one day that even brain surgery feels boring to her sometimes.

Some days, practice is an act of faith, moving *as if* it will help, moving *as if* you want to, moving *as if* you care. The promise is that the *as if* will eventually start to be replaced by *this is part of who I am*. For many people who have been traumatized, believing in the possibility of "eventually" can be the hardest act of faith of all. Having a sense of future can feel like someone else's pipe dream. That is one of the most elusive aspects of trauma—the way it can deny people a sense of future. To ask survivors to act *as if* you are invested or committed can feel like one big charade. For survivors, the future is an unexpected contingency, a state you can't count on or plan for.

But healers tell us that sitting through practice will eventually bring you a sense of future where you won't need to run so fast from your past. Those who have sat themselves into a place of predictability offer a "sky of wisdom" in exchange for the boring, scary frustration of some everyday practices.

When Chaos Is Easier Than Stillness

This is a song for every girl who's
ever been through something
she thought she couldn't make it through.
I sing these words because I was that girl too
wanting something better than this
but who do I turn to?
Now we are moving from the darkness into the light
this is the defining moment of our lives.
    —India.Arie[13]

For trauma survivors, recognizing reasons for gaps in practice can be part of healing itself. This awareness is illustrated in the story of a student of mine, Julia, a thirty-one-year-old white woman who runs a lively and well-respected afterschool program at a community center in Boston. She first practiced yoga at a local gym when she was eighteen. Her first yoga memory was after a class when she was playing one of her favorite hip-hop CDs only to realize that it seemed too intense, too frantic. She was struck by how easily yoga calmed her down and helped her find her breath.

As someone who grew up with parents who were addicted to heroin and grandparents who had drinking problems, this calm was a huge relief. Chaos and inconsistency were the norms in her family along with regularly being told that if she and her siblings acted better, their parents would stop using drugs. Although school provided some respite from the chaos, her community felt unstable because of the nearby casino.

Once she went to college she lost track of yoga as deep depression swallowed her up. When I asked her why she didn't pursue yoga, she explained: "With depression, I felt like a stranger in my own skin. During that time, I didn't want to be around people, particularly those who knew me as happy and focused. So, I isolated myself, spending many days and nights on my couch, afraid to let people see how I really felt."

The next time she tried yoga, about a decade later, she immediately felt a confidence and energy that buoyed her. She loved the postures, and deep breathing lowered her anxiety. When I asked her why it took a decade for her to return to yoga, she explained that for people who grew up with family dysfunction associated with addictions (not paying the bills, frequent moves, divorce) it is hard to do anything that is consistent as an adult. She knew that yoga requires consistency. Plus she had become adept at taking care of other people but had very few skills in taking care of herself. Julia went so far as to set up a yoga program for at-risk girls even though she didn't take yoga classes herself. Yoga felt decadent and somehow not as important as her work with youth.

Now that she is doing yoga again, she is thrilled but worried that she won't be able to sustain it. Each week that she comes feels like a big accomplishment. In just a few months of regular practice, she is finding an inner peace on and off the mat. She finds herself smiling unabashedly after years of covering her face when she smiled. She is also attracting other positive changes in her life, including having met a loving, supportive, and healthy boyfriend. But change, even positive change, can feel scary. When toxicity is the norm in someone's childhood, it is scary to get into a healthy relationship. It is scary to feel seen and respected on the mat. It is scary to know that memories may come up, that she may need to deal with buried pain. Julia says that because of the risk required to maintain a steady practice, teachers "need to applaud our commitment and willingness to show up." It takes determination to get into the room and stay there. Honoring people's progress each day—the little, immediate signs of it—can make a big difference in how people feel about yoga.

A few months ago, Julia was held up on the street when she was walking home from work. When she started to fight back, the man drew a gun. One of Julia's bosses said fighting back showed signs of instability and irrationality, which only added insult to injury. In the past, Julia might have let depression and anger bury her, finding herself drinking on the couch rather than going to yoga. But this time, she came to yoga and then talked about the assault after class. At this point, she is at the edge between believing in yoga and not. She has a close friend who recently earned her yoga certification who Julia has watched gain confidence as she has studied. But fear and ego often stand in Julia's way. And she doesn't feel at all close to clearing her mind when she is practicing. "Maybe," she tells me, "my mind calms a little, but I still wrestle with obsessive thoughts and a lot of anxiety. This is the challenge, making a new life, knowing that I deserve love and support in my work, in my practice, in my relationships." As she tells me, "I can do chaos. I know chaos. It is a whole other thing to say I can do yoga. And I will. That is what I am working on now."

Nine Lives

For trauma survivors, one difficult lesson requires recognizing how many times we need to save our own lives. The first time you did this you might not have even been aware of your courage. Typically, it is more like a gut instinct that takes over—an involuntary impulse. Run out of your house that is on fire, stay low to the ground, take shallow breaths, keep running; or, leave this family as fast as you can, save all of your babysitting money, don't tell people you have it; or, pick up the sleeping baby from her crib in the middle of the night and speed out of the driveway before your husband wakes up. Those are initial "save your life" actions that you might not even know you are taking at the time—it is more like getting the hell out of Dodge.

The next time you save your life might rely less on instinct, more on planning. These times might come because of an external crisis—an illness, death, or assault. What do you need to save your life after chemo and radiation? How can you recreate your life after your partner has died of AIDS? Can you leave that job that is killing those around you and may kill you, too? What steps will help you recover from rape?

In some ways, the second and third life-saving may be easier than the first. You might have more resources, including supportive friends and family, witnesses, a steady income, a certain wisdom that comes with age. But this life-saving can be challenging as well—less driven by an automatic response, more complicated in terms of the necessary steps. This is where tenacity comes into play. You may be around people who don't expect you to save your life. There are so many walking dead, even within our own families, so much permission to just make do after a trauma. (Give him another drink, look the other way when a vet gets addicted to painkillers, don't say anything about a family member who is working eighty hours a week.)

Another stumbling block in staying on the healing path comes from knowing, in your bones, what it took to survive before—a knowledge that can make gearing up feel daunting. You may be more tired from getting out of Dodge before. It may be difficult because a second or third crisis may bring up the first injury or loss. Trauma is like that, sidling up to what came before. The difference between surviving a first life-threatening crisis and subsequent ones can be compared to the difference between getting stung by one wasp and getting stung by a whole swarm, the toxic shock cumulative, overwhelming. There is a reason that many people take issue with the term *post–traumatic stress disorder*. It may not feel like "post" at all, especially if you get hit by another trauma before you have had the chance to recover from the first.

I am reminded of a friend of mine, a longtime yogi, who has had a home practice for decades. Yoga had been central to her healing after multiple losses in her young life. When she decided to move her family from Brazil to Boston temporarily, leaving her husband behind because of his work commitments, she had much to accomplish—finding schools for her children, securing a new job as a choreographer, helping her son with a chronic illness. It took a while for her to find time for the mat again, her daily tasks making practice feel like just one more thing to accomplish. Then her daughter was diagnosed with cancer, and vigils and visits to the hospital became a daily routine. During that time, she spoke fondly of yoga, but getting to the mat felt too exposing, as if she might crumble if she started to stretch out again. As is true for many, the mat became a repository for what felt scary. In this instance, focusing on her life seemed irrelevant in the face of helping her daughter survive. The hide-and-seek of practice requires being patient with what life brings. Seeking the mat again sometimes takes its own time.

This patience is difficult for trauma survivors. We know, firsthand, how precious and vulnerable life is. We also know how trauma costs time—sometimes weeks, months, whole years of our lives. Survivors often live with a deep sense of urgency (which may be a diplomatic way of saying impatience). This is what Pema Chödrön realized when she decided to take vows as a Buddhist nun, even though, in comparison to most, she came to the robing late in life. She said she had some catching up to do, that there was "no time to lose."[14] This sense of urgency can bring people back to yoga, even though doing so can feel like dragging a cranky, scared child there. The mat is good for that—hearing your worries and sadness, as you remember that healing can build on the resilience that has come before.

Sweet Spot

> The Buddha would say that most people throw themselves into the
> river of life and float downstream, moved here and there by the
> current. But the spiritual aspirant must swim upstream, against the
> current of habit, familiarity, and ease.
> —Eknath Easwaran[15]

On first reading, swimming upstream seems to contradict the emphasis
of many yogis on cultivating comfort and ease. Patanjali's oft-cited sutra
explicitly states: "The physical postures should be steady and comfortable."[16] The practice of asanas centers on finding balance and relaxation
in a pose—finding comfort in warrior I pose *(virabhadrasana I),* where
you are low enough to the ground to feel a stretch but not so low that
you pull a hamstring; when you twist tightly enough in eagle pose *(garudasana)* that you can align the joints, feel the steadiness, but not wind up
so tightly that your face is tense and you stop breathing. Finding the sweet
spot is what separates yoga from purely physical exercise and comes from
coordinating the breath with the pose.

Such a commitment hardly sounds like choosing to live the life of a
salmon. And yet, I have often needed to swim upstream—to move beyond
habit and familiarity—to then find ease. I have watched yoga students
need to swim against addictions—cigarettes, alcohol, drugs—and away
from toxic family members. Sometimes they have needed to move to
other states and countries in order to heal. A yogi friend said his move
ten thousand miles from where he was raised was essential to feel his
own breath, to know that yoga and meditation were the right path for
him. Another student said doing double practices, morning and night,
was essential to break her habit of calling her former partner, who had
been abusive. Breaking cycles takes doing things in new ways, creating
pathways for healing.

Recently, when I was walking around Jamaica Pond in Boston, my
friend Peg pointed out a row of circular formations of stones beneath
the water's surface. Having never noticed them before, I was intrigued to

learn they are "fish beds." I had never even thought about what fish do to prepare for laying eggs. It turns out that while salmon swim upstream to lay their eggs, other fish make nests in calm water. With stones, sticks, and other ordinary-extraordinary items available to them, they create havens for regeneration without needing the ordeal of the fateful upstream swim.

The yoga mat is a kind of fish bed. What comforts me about rolling out the mat and placing it in the same sweet spot at the studio day after day is that the mat accommodates me as I alternate between being a salmon and turning around to let the current carry me downstream, each time offering space to find the warm current in between.

Hungry, Angry, Lonely, Tired

> Be patient with your stumbling. Anger goes away if it isn't treated as
> though it is special.
> —Geri Larkin[17]

In *Stumbling Toward Enlightenment,* Geri Larkin tells many stories about
stumbling in her own practice. In one she chronicles when she had a full-
fledged panic attack while accompanying her daughter for a skin cancer
test. As a woman who had taken many risks in her life—surfing, skiing,
skydiving, meditating in caves with bats—Larkin was shocked by her
nausea, sweaty hands, and racing heartbeat. A therapist advised Larkin
that if the symptoms came again, she might try sitting with them, rather
than trying to stop them. When her panic grew the next time her daughter
had an appointment, Larkin sat with it until "Bam! It was gone. For good.
I had put myself in the monster's mouth, climbed into the belly of the
whale, and it was gone. No tranquilizers, no alcohol to numb the fear, no
panic attack or support groups. The fear was gone."[18]

This is where getting to the mat comes in. I have watched people come
through the door looking jumbled and pissed off, but by the time they
leave they look less frantic and less depressed. I have a student who, after
losing his wife to cancer, came to the mat feeling so hurt that his chest
ached. Most days, after class, he reported feeling lighter. I have memories
of surviving a breakup by riding feelings of deep sadness through a practice. Losing that relationship brought up many feelings of abandonment
and loss that, as it turns out, I hadn't dealt with. On the mat, I wrestled
with these emotions, while endorphins and relaxation became welcome
relief. The combination of the comfort of child's pose (balasana), the rising energy in bird of paradise *(svarga dvidasana),* and the reverence of toe
stand (padangustasana) helped me through the loss. Finding alignment
in my body led me toward a sense of equanimity even when the grieving was fierce. I can still see the small Buddha statue at the studio where
I practiced during that time, remembering that the feelings I had when

looking at the Buddha changed over time. Feelings do eventually pass. While they may return, time and practice often soften them.

One of the healing powers of yoga is its ability to help people ride complicated emotions on the mat so they don't overwhelm us after. In twelve-step programs for people who are recovering from addictions, there is an acronym—HALT—for hungry, angry, lonely, and tired. These are four states that, left unchecked, are likely to lead people to use (food and drugs). The idea is to address these states as soon as they arise—call a sponsor; eat healthy meals so that we can put food away between meals; find ways to cope with anger; try to avoid pushing too hard (with work, in relationships) that leave little or nothing left for self-care. The longer we travel into the land of hungry, angry, lonely, or tired, the harder it can be to find a way back to a sense of ease and equanimity.

One step away from the hungry-angry-lonely-tired litany includes bringing the states to the mat. Yoga can intercept HALT and transform these emotions. Such a practice often takes time, requires what may seem like an impossible state—patience. Larkin says, "Be patient with your stumbling." I know I am a stumbler. Getting to the studio can break the isolation that many survivors struggle with. In this case, practicing twists and straddles with a partner or balancing stick and petal pose in a circle can be an emblem for our willingness to reach beyond HALT and toward each other.

From Stone to Sand to Water

Patterns of behavior and emotions are etched into our minds in one of three ways—as lines in water, lines in sand, and lines in stone.[19] Trauma survivors first come to the mat with many patterns etched in stone. Over time, the etchings can start to soften—become lines of sand, and then, eventually, lines of water as you swim around much more freely, much less tied down than when you were operating through patterns of stone. Typically, there is no formal sign announcing these changes since they tend to be subtle. And it is difficult to see the changes in ourselves. We are too close to have that perspective.

Healing can feel elusive, often giving the feeling that you might not be progressing even when you are. There are many reasons for this. First, the most important work is being done underground, in your nervous system, in your lymph system, in your mind. It is easy to miss the work as it is happening. It's a little bit like the work involved in fixing a house. When people buy a fixer-upper, oftentimes the most expensive jobs are the plumbing and electrical work. You can spend thousands of dollars on that work, but because almost all of the work is inside of the walls, you can't see it.

A second reason change is difficult to measure is because as you get more sophisticated in your poses and meditation, the adjustment and concentration will need to be finer. The more subtle the concentration, the more concentrated the mind needs to become. There is a big difference, for example, between the first time you are able to stay for a whole practice (without having to leave out of fear or feeling flooded emotionally) and the more minute process of staying focused on your breath through an entire sequence. You can see the person flying out of the room (especially if that person is you), while gauging whether a person is breathing deeply is harder to recognize. You might not even know yourself. It's a more subtle adjustment. But that difference is a huge sign of progress that may manifest in not bolting from a healthy relationship—learning how to read someone's expressions, being able to weather the ups and downs of time together.

For people who have been scared by emotions of any kind—anger, jealousy, fear, rage, shame, sadness—it can take a while to move from not knowing what you are feeling to accepting that feelings are temporary, that they come and go. Another step is accepting a range of emotions—some from before, some from the present, many complicated. This challenge is one reason some trauma survivors get stuck in the land of all-angry, the land of all-sad, or of all-worry. One feeling, even if it is scary, can feel easier than being barraged by a range of emotions. Another step is being able to name multiple feelings, all at once, and then, with work, letting them go, too. For many people, a flowing yoga sequence is especially helpful in learning to ride emotions, getting used to easing in and out of postures, letting sensations and feelings wash over you as you practice.

Like a Kite with No String

Part of why healing from trauma can seem erratic is because of the emotional, psychic, and spiritual walls that we hit—and that we often don't see in front of us. One of my biggest walls had to do with meditation. This was an embarrassing wall for me, partly because meditation is integral to corpse pose (savasana), the culminating pose in most yoga practices. While I had been in a variety of meditation circles since my mid-twenties, it wasn't until I had been doing an asana practice consistently for a number of years that I could get quiet and experience stillness.

Posture sequences taught in a set order each time eased me into meditation by allowing me to let a range of sensations come through me— pain, fear, joy, exhilaration, exhaustion—in a controlled way, one posture at a time, with a rest in between. So that, as the sensations came up, I knew that they were time-specific. Years of learning and feeling these sensations come and go, rise and then fall, helped me with meditation, starting to learn that feelings come and go, too.

Once I could see feelings as temporary, I could also begin to understand what meditators refer to as letting go of story. For a long time, this concept scared me. Meditators seemed to talk about it as a place of consciousness beyond emotion and ego. In her profound book, *Radical Acceptance*, Tara Brach wrote a passage about this that has followed me, insisting that I listen: "Each time we let go of our story, we realize that there is no ground to stand on, no position that orients us, no way to hide or avoid what is arising."[20] When I first read that quote, I thought, why would I deliberately seek a psychic state that did not include language? Words are what I held onto when I was young, words at the bottom of coloring-book pages. Words and writing have been how I feel like I exist. They ground me to the earth, to people. I asked myself, why would I deliberately make time during my day to find a place beyond words—a place that to me felt like being a kite with no string? What kind of crazy person would do that? That would be nuts.

This was one of my walls. It took me a long time to understand that a space beyond story and explanation is like looking at the stars, feeling small, but also part of a larger universe at the same time. My guess is that the many years of asana along with my stubborn willingness to try meditation, give up on it, and then try again finally opened a way for me to experience quiet and aloneness that wasn't so scary and lonely. This experience then opened up a whole range of yoga practices that before I thought were boring, or just too quiet for someone like me.

Somewhere along the way in my mad quest to not let meditation intimidate me, I consulted my then ninety-nine-year-old grandmother. By that point, she was spending entire days in her reclining chair, from when she woke up until she went to sleep. As she described it, she spent most of her time floating, her mind like a sea anemone, dancing with the tide, inside the rhythm of water. Increasingly she was going deep inside, to an interior place where there was little fear, anger, or worry. As she shared with me, it occurred to me she was talking about an awareness that many meditators describe that had been threatening to me. Somehow, I began to understand that the groundlessness she was talking about was leading her to new ground, one that connects us not to our physical bodies or to our emotions or our reactions or our stories, but to our connectedness to each other, to the earth, to breath, to light.

In and Out of Time

Let me wear the day
Well so when it reaches you
You will enjoy it.
—Sonia Sanchez[21]

Sonia Sanchez wrote this poem when she was in China, thinking about her twin sons in Philadelphia who would be waking thirteen hours after her. I have always thought of time as mysterious—time here is not time there, morning is night and night is morning. The orbit of the earth around the sun speaks to the relativity of time, a human construct that meditators teach us does not exist as we imagine. A minute can feel like a day, a day like an hour, certain moments lasting so long—the last gaze before the train door shuts, the time it took me to move down the stairs (will it be forever?) to open the screen door that had closed on my oldest dog's tail, her eyes pleading.

The in and out of time teaches us lessons on the mat: some days practice squeaks by like an old refrigerator, bones cold and brittle; other days the flow picks me up and I ride on a carpet ride of breath. Time moves forward and back, reminding us not to get dragged out by a creaky, sad hour. Patanjali wrote, "When the mind has settled, we are established in our true nature, which is unbounded consciousness."[22] In this state, time is not stuck. Freedom is a natural seat in this space. Inhale and exhale guides. Time is not what it seems. We are all capable of more than we know now, waiting for the sun to come to us from the east.

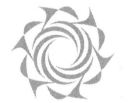

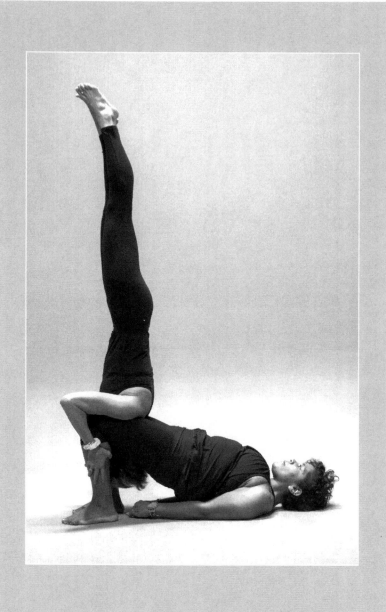

PART IV

The Color of Rothko's Blue

Long-Term Wholeness

One of the promises of long-term yoga is its ability to open us to the deeper dimensions of yoga, including the expansion of consciousness. As awareness of our life force (prana) expands, our sense of our potential grows in tandem. Such awareness can include seeing your body as a source of insight and a "vehicle for perception."[1] Tapping into what yogis refer to as your "energetic body" can allow access to new knowledge and powers of healing, the recognition of other people's vital energy, and connection to energy in nature. The energetic body is considered one of the five koshas, or layers of the soul, that also include the physical, mental, wise, and bliss body. Yoga functions to create balance among these layers while opening us to their powers. Many stories in this section attest to development of the energetic body as a key component of long-term healing.

Accessing this energetic awareness can be exhilarating—a kind of jolt to the senses that occurs when one reaches a higher plane of consciousness, as I describe in the piece "Urdhvakundalini." But living with this consciousness is not always easy. While part of us may celebrate this energy, another part of us may find ourselves retreating back into an unhealthy relationship, gobbling too much chocolate, or seeking out or even creating drama at work. Sustaining a long-term practice asks us to consider daily ways to work with energy—to channel that energy in positive ways. Deeper access to energy can enhance memory often lost to trauma and its aftermath, which can add calm and confidence to your life.

Long-term healing also includes *svadhyaya*, the Sanskrit word for self-study. The first time I heard the word, I found myself rolling it around on my tongue in delight since it sounds something like getting your *ya-yas* out. The Sanskrit word makes the discipline of self-reflection sound fun, like memorizing the text of the Yoga Sutras while playing on a jungle gym. It's good that the word sounds fun because in reality, the process can be hard work. Self-reflection is required to keep a practice alive and growing. It can take many forms: studying yoga philosophy and history, doing deep work in therapy, meditating, and seeking out the guidance of a master teacher. Whatever path you take, to practice svadhyaya means focusing on the expansion of your interior life, seeking to understand the workings of your own mind.

The growing link between the world of science and the realm of contemplation is a particularly twenty-first-century practice of svadhyaya; it's where study of the mind and energy on the mat meet scientific measurements of brain waves in an MRI. Much of what yogis have long known about the energetic components of yoga is what neuroscientific research on brain integration is now confirming with its brain scans. We have the Dalai Lama to thank for this cross-pollination, because he spearheaded the effort to have neuroscientists study the brain waves of meditators. This century's yoga practitioners who explore svadhyaya ask many complex questions: about sexuality and ethics, ways to solve conflict in an age of unprecedented violence, and what the Buddhist concept of "emptiness" might have to offer people on a healing path.

Along with a commitment to svadhyaya and tuning in to the energetic body, trauma survivors find that our long-term yoga often leads us to other creative activities—dance, music, poetry, writing, painting—that both rewire our brains and open our hearts. Being in that creative space requires us to crawl inside of the unconscious, to get comfortable with the surprises that are there. When I am trying to write a poem, I need to drop down into a contemplative, questioning, vulnerable space where much that is unexpected often lives. This is the brain space where repressed memory, unexplored emotion, and fragments of trauma live. And this is also where joy often lives—where laughter comes from, a surprising new insight, the ability to see a color in a new way. This is also the capacity that can make our hearts expand. I have long thought that the space my drumming friend and former lover Cornell Coley slips into when playing Afro-Cuban rhythms with his band connects to the calm and focused attention I see on his face when he is practicing yoga. Long-term practice has the ability to help us live as fully as possible, to find talents that might have been forgotten or postponed.

It is also no surprise that long-term yoga may also bring changes in our relationship to our physical practice. While early yoga often centers on a physical practice, later yoga often draws more deeply on meditation and spiritual awakening. As Richard Miller, a leader in yoga therapy, writes, "In 1976 I was practicing the King Dancer's Pose, holding my leg behind my head while standing balanced on the opposite leg. I asked myself, 'What have I attained after so much effort?' I realized that were I to walk out the door and be hit by a car, the flexibility I had gained would be worthless. At that moment, I realized that the goal of hatha yoga had to be more than the attainment of some perfected body position. And that has been true ever since."[2]

The consciousness that long-term practice can nurture speaks to my own predilection for a variety of approaches to wholeness. This multi-dimensionality is what you can see in the color of blue in many of Mark Rothko's paintings, a blue that actually contains multiple shades of brown as well. You can see this layering of beauty in the span of the dancers' arms in Alvin Ailey's signature piece, *Revelations*. You can feel it in the poetry of Rumi and Pablo Neruda, Joy Harjo and Nâzim Hikmet. Through experiencing the expansion of consciousness that yoga promises, we can feel this creativity and power in ourselves, and incite it, one yoga posture at a time.

Urdhvakundalini

A few years ago, at the end of an intense yoga class in Bali, I sensed an overwhelming wave of energy flowing through me as soon as the teacher put on a chant to accompany us in corpse pose (savasana). The energy was so strong that I sat straight up and walked to the back of the room. Then, for what was less than fifteen minutes but seemed timeless, I felt waves of grief, a sensation that led me to lift my arms and begin to cradle what felt like the earth in my hands. As I stood, I was profoundly moved by both the beauty and fragility of the earth, and all of her sentient creatures. I deeply understood that life is both fleeting and enduring, that the life force, the prana, recycles through endless generations, continually renewing itself. Once the music was over and the practice ended, I knew that I would never forget that experience. I had been simultaneously grief-stricken and joyful, and it seemed to be telling me that my work in the world, my dharma, was about recognizing this—this paradox that I had held in my hands. This experience also reassured me about my dharma as a teacher and writer, both commitments done in community.

This kind of experience may last for a short period of time, but the lesson or feeling that resides within it can stay with you for a lifetime. It is like riding a bike. Once you know how, the knowledge never leaves you. This moment of pure awareness, which may come as quickly as it goes, is what yogis refer to as *urdhvakundalini*—the rising of energy through a median channel of the body that unfolds energy and consciousness.[3] It is a moment of feeling connected with infinity, a luminous experience beyond the ego, beyond the normal limits humans face in our days. This is what the word "yoga" means—union—with higher states of consciousness, creating an expansive connection to the world.

Yoga can help you hear your inner wisdom. Over time, you know better what work you are meant to do in the world. You know better your passions and purpose, your special and unique gifts. Wisdom is more than intelligence. It is more than making good decisions. It is speaking from the inside out rather than from the outside in, being able to draw upon your lived experience to make decisions that will help you grow rather than stay stuck. This wisdom comes from your own essence—not from your spouse, or family, or a religious institution, or the media.

While the specific physical and mental gifts that come from yoga vary for each person, many of them are identifiable, some even visually. Those that are less concrete, and take place at the level of the energetic body, can be even more transformative. As you keep practicing, you will likely experience spontaneous moments of union with a spirit or energy that transcends thought. This energetic body helps you discern what is actually going on in situations that don't make sense on a rational plane. This power allows you to tap into your intuitive powers and arrive at solutions you might not otherwise see. It enables you to sense your internal organs and know what you need to heal yourself, with far greater wisdom than your rational mind possesses, and long before a doctor might be able to help.

Signs of access to your energetic body may manifest themselves in fleeting and unanticipated ways. But when they do show up, the core truth of this energy can be convincing at a level that goes deeper than words.

Life on the Thirty-Sixth Floor

In a dharma talk, Kripalu teacher Devadas Day used an analogy of climbing to the top of a thirty-six-floor apartment building to explain the heightened consciousness that long-term yoga can create.[4] Normally, Day said, he lives on the tenth floor. This is the level where he feels competent, focused, and able to be present with others. When he dips below the tenth floor, life seems like a struggle, he's easily frustrated, and he isn't available to the people in his life. So, he does what he needs to do to stay on the tenth floor.

One of the gifts of yoga, though, is its ability to help him climb up to the higher floors, all the way up to the thirty-sixth floor. This is the level of heightened creativity where he feels a transcendent energetic connection to consciousness.

The challenge of rising to the thirty-sixth floor, however, is that if you are used to existing on the tenth floor, you may not feel comfortable as you start to climb. It may seem unstable and scary. That is why it often happens that as soon as we access the energies of the thirty-sixth floor, many of us revert to activities that will pull us back down—a box of cookies, a drink, the TV, a destructive relationship—all energy drains rather than enhancers. But over time, as you keep up your practice, and as you start spending more time on higher floors, yoga allows you to get increasingly comfortable on the thirty-sixth floor, to experience it as a place that is not only exalted but safe.

Being on the thirty-sixth floor also allows you to see the world from a new perspective. If you imagine that the thirty-six-story building is next to a park, you can visualize how different the view of that park is when looked at from the first floor as opposed to the tenth and how vastly different it will look from the top floor. The actual park has not changed, just your perspective on it.

Understanding the potential to make this shift is important for survivors. Over time, as you climb higher, you alter how you respond to the triggers that revive your experience of trauma. And when you learn how to stay steady in the face of those triggers, you will see the trauma from a different perspective. You will be able to stay in your thirty-sixth-story perch, looking down at the trauma from a safe distance, high on the energy of life—your own endless supply of prana.

So, the next time you get scared by being up on the thirty-sixth floor, first try to have a little compassion for yourself. Old behaviors, particularly those triggered by a freeze-and-submit response at the level of the parasympathetic nervous system, are difficult to break. Zoning out in front of the TV, eating or drinking too much, withdrawing from people, running away from challenges—these are all examples of the old behaviors you might have fallen into when you didn't have a choice, before you learned how to step back and observe. But now, instead of acting on impulse and reaching for that drink, or brownie, or connection to someone who is more stuck than you, remember that you have choices. You can try popping into a headstand cycle (sirsasana) for a few minutes and then see how you feel. Or try doing ten sun salutations (surya namaskar) with your eyes closed, slowly following the breath with each movement. And then check in. Or, try doing a Vinyasa Flow series at a neighborhood park with your best playlist as company, coordinating your savasana with Dianne Reeves or Snatam Kaur or another musician who inspires you.

The Energy within the Postures

At the center of developing a consciousness of collective belonging and creativity is grounding ourselves with our breath. In another dharma talk, Devadas Day addressed why breath is crucial for opening the energetic body. Devadas talks about this work as developing out of a thousand years of interlacing connections between tantra (ancient meditation techniques for spiritual expansion) and alchemy (a philosophical tradition linking science with magic). People who practiced tantra and alchemy were interested in rituals and visualizations that could work with energy to generate internal transformation. By the time hatha yoga emerged (around 1000 CE), an increasing number of poses were being discovered and practiced that, like the earlier rituals and visualizations, worked with energy.

This history is important for trauma survivors because our healing includes gaining access to energy from inside and around us. The people who practiced tantra, alchemy, and later, hatha yoga all believed that the body held keys to energy transformation—that the body is a location for liberation. This, I know, is a tricky concept, since for many people the very site we are now looking to as a source of liberation is the same location where so much damage was done. The good news, though, is that this healing practice is ancient. We don't need to create these methods of healing from scratch. By practicing yoga we are attaching ourselves to a long line of healers.

Devadas Day talks about how, as you consistently practice, you will start to see that while the physical postures matter, what is more important is the energy inside of them. The analogy Devadas gives is of a frying pan you are using to make tofu pups (hot dogs without the meat). While you need the pan, what matters is the energy the tofu pup will provide, its taste, its texture, its length, its color. That is the same with the energy of a pose—learning to pay attention to the sensation inside of the container, inside the posture. That doesn't mean you can just start doing whatever you want. Holding onto certain forms still matters. But more important than what a pose looks like is how you feel (and the energy you can sense) as you go inside the pose.

This distinction between the frying pan and the tofu pup, between the poses and the energy inside, means you get a chance every day to notice the sensations inside your body, knowing that they are protected by form—the shape of the pose itself. That's the beauty about practicing poses. Unlike with meditation, where it is not clear where your mind might take you, your body has biological stops that will only let you go so far at first and, sometimes, for years. Your body is a natural container that has limits and borders. That is why it is important not to push too hard—to be patient and gentle. That is one way you can trust your body. Your hamstrings will tell you when not to stretch any farther in seated forward bend (paschimottanasana); your sacrum will tell you, if you are listening, when to back off in wind removing pose *(pavanamuktasana)*. The pose is the container holding the energy. This energy will change, grow, and become more distinct and revealing with time. As you start to respect your limits, the edges of the frying pan, you will be able to key into the energy going on inside of it.

Paying attention to the energetic body, not just the external pose, is what yogis refer to as shifting from approaching yoga as a willful practice, to one that is based in breath and ease. This becomes important for those who try extra hard, who think they are not enough, not ever right. I am not saying that yoga isn't strenuous. But the strenuousness can still come from a place of relaxing into the sensations that, over time, get friendlier. It is like imagining that you are an eagle scanning a valley, a turtle taking in sun, a loon measuring depth, a flamingo in tree pose.

Open the Channels

The goal of yoga
is to open the channels and undo the blocks
prepare for meditation

Gaining access to new awareness can be among the most profound gifts of a devoted yoga practice. This gift can come in many forms, including the ability to channel insight through the body. A few years ago I attended a writer's conference that included a session where writers spoke about channeling portions of their poetry, novels, and essays.[5] The intimacy in the room as they began to speak let me know this sharing was unplanned. There is still enough stigma and mystery about channeling knowledge that you could feel the risk-taking in the room.

When I first channeled words onto the page, I felt shy and nervous about talking about it. Several years previously, I had written a memoir about the first year of living with my adopted son, LaMar.[6] This book had written itself like none of my others. I witnessed complete chapters come through me, almost verbatim, once every two or three weeks, for nine months. The impulse to write was so strong that sometimes I needed to pull my car over to the side of the road, slip out of meetings, or get up in the middle of the night to write.[7]

Channeled writing is different from other writing. The contrast between the intimacy, ease and power of this creative process and the more straightforward linear writing I am most familiar with is why I pray for more visitations, the experience of writing with a channel magical, more communal than other writing. Long-term yoga practice can open creative channels. Sometimes, this access makes me nervous, but mostly it makes me excited.

In my situation, I had been doing yoga for many years before I sought guidance from a somatic therapist who helped me work with memories stuck in my body that, once released, brought me new awareness. It was during this therapy that I experienced overwhelming body memories of having been strangled under water when I was very young. As is often true for early trauma, my memory of it is incoherent and fragmented. It came in the form of a seizure, starting below my right shoulder and then coming through my neck, up through the top of my head. It felt like a fat snake wiggling itself up and out of my body. The therapist witnessed this ritual movement during four sessions. If someone had described such a process to me, I might have thought to myself—"Yep, a little bit crazy"— had I not experienced it myself.

A gift from this work was that the release cleared a channel that had been blocked. I discovered that the ache I had felt was about people and places I had lost as well as from not yet having access to spirits and knowledge coming through me. It was as if the radio station of this consciousness was inside me all along, but I didn't know how to tune into the right station, to hear the sound. It is like sensing that there is beautiful music playing nearby but not being able to find the music festival (and constantly "forgetting" that it is possible to hear the music at all).

Gaining access to that channel may follow the spiritual death that trauma first evokes. It may be hard to talk about trauma as a spiritual death—it sounds so dramatic, so drastic. At least temporarily, trauma kills a sense of innocence. Early trauma can sabotage whole developmental phases that, once missed, are very hard to make up for later in life. Trauma jerry-rigs the lymphatic and nervous system and can leave one feeling jumpy, literally and figuratively, for a long time. This all can add up to losing a faith in human goodness, in a belief that the earth is a safe place, a fear of trusting people, and a willingness to take risks, even safe ones. These are symptoms that show us that healing needs to happen at the level of the body and the mind, in the lymph system and at the level of the spirit—and that all these are interrelated. Our bodies have remarkable abilities to regenerate themselves. This regeneration initiates a whole series of spiritual awakenings from places we might never have named. In the process, trauma survivors can become company to each other, fluttering above psychic graveyards, very much *in* this world.

On the night after the conference panel with the writers who talked about channeling, I went back to my room to practice yoga only to find myself resisting, fear lapping around my edges, and then an overwhelming feeling that I needed to close my eyes. Then I heard this directive that I interpreted as a communal message:

Close your eyes. That is where the knowledge is. The space standing between you and the channel that will guide you is your fear that loneliness will envelop you, smother you if you go inside. Your fear of shutting your eyes is standing in the way of direct communication with a multicolored channel. The channel is the link to your own spirit. It may not be an actual person. It may be a presence, in the form of colors. This awareness will find its way through music; will find it through dance. Walk outside of the lines now. You need to do some of that walking alone. There will be others on this path whom you don't know yet. Pare down. Hone down. Simplify. The easiest access will be in early morning. Let the morning have space for this creativity.

Of the many yoga traditions currently available to us, Kundalini Yoga may be the most explicit in identifying how yoga can stimulate creative energy. Practicing Kundalini *kriyas* (a set of exercises) in tandem with painting, dancing, writing, and other creative work can bring forth surprising, original work that highlights our interconnection to other sentient beings and the world.[8] This creativity may be especially useful for trauma survivors for whom the trauma included feeling trapped, blocked, clipped, or alone as we uncover essential and vital capacities. Finding portals into new creativity returns us to what Kundalini teachers refer to as "Source"—that is infinitely creative, wise, and regenerative. The Source can remind us of our deepest selves (our soul) and our connection to each other. Recovering body memories through asana and then translating these memories into art is a powerful way to link the rational to the magical to transform what was stuck into beauty, into life. That is what doing yoga and making art can do, as survivors celebrate our creativity, discover new realms.

Steadiness of Mind

While all of the limbs of yoga work with energy, the sixth, dharana, is especially relevant when it comes to learning to fine-tune energy. Dharana is often described in a shorthand way as concentration, although as Yoga Sutra translator Alistair Shearer has noted, Patanjali was actually talking about something deeper than that. The promise of dharana is that "the longer the mind can remain effortlessly focused while in a state of relaxation, the more powerful it becomes."[9] Patanjali didn't mean "powerful" in the Tonka truck, corporate mogul, most-guns-in-the-world connotation of the word. He meant a power that allows you to feel comfortable in your skin: that finds you among people and trees and oceans that inspire you; a willingness to be simultaneously tough and vulnerable, contained and expansive.

A key characteristic I have seen among long-term yogis is an ability to develop dharana on and off the mat. This relaxed steadiness can be seen when what seems like "scattered pieces start to gather."[10] It is when you look up from the desk after writing, thinking it has been fifteen minutes when it has been an hour, your mind connecting your world-words together on the page. It can be when you see that the iridescent green on the newly grown spring fern coming out of the rock is the rock and the rock is the fern. It occurs before you catch yourself aware of this knowledge. It can be listening to the tone of a cello in all of its resonance carrying the string's life force as part of the wood's base sound, knowing that the sound, the string, the wood and your listening are all one object.

Steadiness of mind is what allows people on a healing path to stay in your own reality when the world around you feels like it is spinning out of control. It is the ability to stay inside the music, inside your breath during practice even as the person next to you starts to flap her mat and fix her hair. Steadiness of mind allows you to walk by a jackhammer and stay in tune with your companion, in step with her stride, even as the jackhammer reminds you of the sound of bullets pummeling the streets in your neighborhood. That steadiness doesn't mean ignoring the jackhammer and its associations. It means being able to talk about it, and then return to the quiet inside of you, a bubble surrounding you and your companion as you walk.

No Center, No Periphery

In the Yoga Sutras, Patanjali links concentration (dharana) with meditation (dhyana) and bliss (samadhi)—considering them collectively as a
state of "perfect discipline" *(samyama)*. Samyama allows people to "experience limitless knowledge and powers, such as the ability to know past
and future, enter into other bodies, and understand the languages of
animals and birds."[11] It can be scary at first to talk about these experiences.
I have worried people will think I am making them up, or boasting. Or
that identifying these experiences out loud might make them disappear.
And yet, naming the experiences can help us better understand dynamics for expanded consciousness. I have a friend who, after about a decade
of yoga, began to sense fields of flowers, rolling hills and cows inside her
spine when her energetic body was open. Her sense was that she was the
flowers, the hills, and the cows, and they were her.

You might rightfully ask why it would be useful for people to experience flowers and hills and cows inside them? Why might sensing others'
bodies bring one to a sense of peace? According to many yogis, psychologists, and mystics, we are born into the world knowing how to do this—it
is part of our birthright. But much that goes on in the world begins to
make such an integration and connection frightening. It can feel scary
for sexual abuse survivors to cultivate an awareness of our connection
to other human bodies because it might remind us of the blurring of
boundaries during a violation. Why does it make any sense to feel our
connection to others' bodies if that might include the bodies of people
who hurt us? Isn't one of the most difficult consequences of trauma a
lost ability to see ourselves as separate from the perpetrator? To carry the
perpetrator's guilt and shame around with us as if it is ours? These are
hard questions. We all deserve a life free of the guilt, shame, disgust, pity,
and confusion that actually belong to those who harmed us.

This is the thing: if one of the consequences of trauma was taking on
the emotions, thoughts, and actions of the perpetrator—not being able
to separate his or her experiences from ours—healing involves recognizing that ability in us. We already have a previous experience, albeit a

frightening, overwhelming one, of seeing ourselves in another, of being entangled with other. This is knowledge that we can now turn toward channeling, sensing, elegantly tuning in with other beings, bodies, animals, trees, the ocean. Yoga can help people fine-tune an invitation into interconnectedness. As longtime yogi Donna Farhi writes, "when we arrive in this place, we realize there is no center and no periphery, that we are in fact infinite and limitless."[12] This is a promise of concentration, meditation, and pure contemplation.

Exquisitely Attuned

Part of what intrigues me about the deeper dimensions of yoga is how they uncover the dialectical nature of trauma; they have the seeds of their own transformation within them. The journey of Arsalan, a psychotherapist, meditator, and dancer friend of mine, gives a marvelous example of this dynamic. As a child Arsalan was painfully shy. He felt deeply disconnected from other people and himself. He spent much of his childhood trying to be invisible, cowering in the face of his emotionally abusive, overpowering father. He also felt like an outsider as a Pakistani Muslim immigrant living in Canada. He wore glasses that he thought contributed to not connecting with people, which is why, once he was old enough, he had eye surgery to correct his vision. The surgery did little to help him feel bonded with people while significantly diminishing his eyesight. While this loss meant he couldn't keep working in information technology, it did eventually lead him to become a psychotherapist, which retrospectively helped him find his dharma, his life's work.

His journey illustrates ways that trauma contains its own methods for healing. The emotional trauma that Arsalan links with hiding behind his glasses is also linked to the path he took to become a therapist. The dynamic of feeling invisible when he was a child is also what makes him exquisitely attuned to ways that clients feel invisible in their own lives. He is transforming the energy of exclusion into energy for healing. The extra work he has needed to do visually is what lets him pay particular attention to how his clients use their eyes in therapy—when they look away, when they look at him, when they drop their gaze. "The hypervigilance that I developed as a child," Arsalan explains, "which is a response to the danger I felt around my father, helped me survive. Many abuse survivors are attuned to body language. So I was not only trying to become invisible by melting into the background, but also was developing ways to protect myself, such as becoming very aware of other people's energy."

Arsalan's commitment to svadhyaya is a crucial aspect of his work. His years practicing meditation, including living in a Buddhist monastery, allowed him to separate his negative thinking from his essence, to create a sense of self that was not based on his father's worldview. Arsalan's sensitivity to his clients carries its own lessons of self-study. To this day, when a client looks away from Arsalan, he initially thinks that he caused his client to avert his or her gaze. Recurrent self-blame requires him to be ever vigilant about how his own patterns still get triggered as a therapist.

His self-reflection also enabled him to find his own idiosyncratic steps toward wholeness. This path has included moving beyond the expectations he was handed growing up Muslim in Pakistan, where stepping out of one's spiritual tradition is considered blasphemy. Such questioning allows him to help clients question their own cultural views. Arsalan says, "Our conditioning as humans is strongly influenced by our parents, culture, and gender. It was liberating for me not to take my cultural views for granted, to be able to pick and choose between what I grew up with and the Western culture I found myself in." Meditation helps with his own questioning, which then helps him as a therapist. He tells me, "I am less triggered by clients' anger, less likely to identify with my own fear, more trusting in the goodness of others, and more able to join people in their own emotional journeys without mixing up my emotional stuff in theirs."

Self-reflection has also taught him to lean into the fear related to the trauma itself. Arsalan tells me, "For a long time I had a fear of older men. So in improvisational dance I would deliberately dance with older men. Similarly, I had a fear of losing control, so I would put myself in dances where I didn't know what the end result would be. In therapy, too, many times you don't know where the discussion is going. It is like jumping off a cliff with a client." His own healing has taught him a clear sense of boundaries and respect for deep listening. He explains, "letting myself go inward—through meditation, therapy, improvisational dancing—all has taken me down a path of healing, for me as well as for those who allow me to walk alongside them as they heal."

Yoga Taught Me Pause

Sometimes, the best way to see the deeper dimensions of yoga comes through in everyday ways. This reality is poignantly illustrated in the life of Patrick, a long-term yoga practitioner, who lives and works in upstate New York. Patrick is deeply respectful of yoga, not in any party-line way but because of how important it has been for him during the past decade. As he said, "Without yoga, I would have lost my mind. Not in a good way as they talk about in yoga. Losing my mind in terms of being dysfunctional. I don't want to be melodramatic, but when I found yoga I was in a very bad place in my life." On the surface, everything looked good. He had five wonderful children and a loving wife. His wife taught at a wealthy college, which meant the family had access to a beautiful campus and free classes, including yoga. He had a respected job as a high school math teacher. As he said, "I had no right to complain. But inside, I was lost and upset. I was getting old and beating up on myself. I wasn't as physically strong any more even though my mind seems sharper and sharper. I was having trouble getting along with one of my children and I could not stop worrying, about everything."

His internal struggles came to a head when he was building a dormer in their house and got caught for doing the construction without a permit. He felt embarrassed and ashamed in a way he couldn't shake. In piecing together why he reacted so strongly to this event, Patrick realized that his working-class Irish Catholic parents' expectations led him to feel great angst about being anything other than perfect. As a child, if he didn't succeed, his parents would tell him, "We don't know what we can say to God about why we failed you." Those expectations translated to his trying to succeed in every way and also sent him crashing when he did not follow his parents' wishes. The story that became emblematic of this occurred after Patrick was working as a civil engineer. He hated his job. His boss was a womanizer, and the company was doing offshore drilling and work for nuclear power plants, all of which Patrick despised. So he quit. When his parents found out, they disowned him, refusing to have any contact with him for years, telling him that he was a disgrace to the family. With this break, Patrick felt tremendous shame.

Once he found yoga he began to find a way out of the perfection vise. He realized that the slower he moved in and out of postures, the more present and alive he felt. It took him five years to do a headstand (sirsasana), a time frame that as a competitive athlete, he couldn't imagine tolerating before. When he landed the posture and dismounted smoothly, his confidence increased. And for the first time, the many things that he intellectually knew he should be proud of he genuinely felt inside as well.

These lessons began to translate off the mat, particularly in his relationships. As a math teacher, he was able to worry less about his students and feel more joy in his work. Yoga has also taught him more about listening. He is someone who has been able to sense people's pain since he was young, a capability that has always helped him as a teacher. With yoga, though, that capability increased. He now knows that when people come to talk with him, his first response can be to step back and relax. He lets them take the lead. As he says, "Yoga has taught me pause."

Yoga also guided him in his relationship with family members to the point where, when he misses yoga for a couple of days in a row, someone will push him out the door, knowing how much calmer and more patient he is with practice. Yoga also gave him structure and ritual when his mother died. When he heard that she was about to pass, he flew to Florida, only to arrive fifteen minutes late. As someone who had heard that a person's spirit stays with her for at least three days after the last breath, Patrick decided to stay and, over the next several days, do as many things as he could that they used to do together. Healing during this mourning period centered on a daily yoga class with an instructor who immediately picked up on Patrick's grieving. Although they spoke very little, her empathetic sensitivity helped Patrick with his initial guilt about not being there the moment his mother died. At another yoga class he attended, the instructor massaged Patrick's face, under his eyes and around his cheeks. With that touch, Patrick felt a big release, as if he was letting go of the grief, at peace with himself and his mother's passing.

Yoga has also taught Patrick to let go of shame, particularly sexual shame carried from growing up with a mother that he intuitively knew had been violated sexually. Yoga has helped him feel more comfortable sexually, to know in his heart the beauty of making love with his wife, particularly when it is with the intention of bringing a child into the world. For Patrick, the two most intimate acts available to people are being present during the birth of one's own child and at the point of death. He believes that corpse pose (savasana) gives people a way to rehearse that letting go. He also sees many parallels between yoga practice and making love. With both, you come alive, get grounded, find release, and then let go. Death is like both making love and savasana, except that when you die, you don't get up the last time.

Long-term yoga has also put Patrick in touch with moments of enlightenment, blips of ineffable expansiveness and peace that he had experienced with LSD in his early twenties. While he had thrilling hallucinations and connections to the "essence" of things, he realized that an essential problem with drugs is that people believe it is not possible to achieve enlightenment without an external substance (that can also cause bodily harm). Yoga, on the other hand, enables a path to enlightenment that rests inside each of us, that we all can find, individually and in community.

Brahmacharya

But what I need is quite specific
terrifying rough stuff and terrific
I need an absolutely one to one a seven-day kiss
—June Jordan[13]

In her essay "I Always Belonged to God," Rama Berch, the originator of Svaroopa Yoga writes about how her sexuality changed as she grew deeper into her practice. She writes, "every morning I got up before the sun—and before my three children awoke—and meditated for an hour. As soon as I sat down, the heat of kundalini climbed up my spine and moved me into fantastic yoga poses." But here is the rub. Berch continues, "I quickly found that if my partner and I had been sexually active the night before, there was no heat, there were no poses—and there was no bliss." This realization led Berch to a practice of celibacy that she writes "has taught me more about relationship than anything else ever had. I have never felt that I was giving something up; I was getting so much more on the inside."[14]

The practice of *brahmacharya*, which has variously been translated as sexual abstinence, sexual moderation, and impeccable sexual behavior, gives yogis a chance to consider this. To not see being sexual as an inevitable rite of passage. To not see sex as the ultimate path to intimacy between two adults. At the same time, for many people who have been sexually abused, finding a way to have beautiful and loving sex can be a crucial way of coming home and completing a cycle of healing, of taking back what was stolen. The complexities of sexuality may be why Patanjali included brahmacharya among the five laws of life (the fourth yama). How we channel sexual energy is crucial, particularly when it comes to something as beautiful and magical, delicate and confusing, essential and divinely inspired as sex.

In this society, confusion about sexuality may begin with how it has been cheapened in this age of pornography, instant intimacy, and the epidemic of sexual violence. The poet and activist Audre Lorde resists this reduction by making a distinction between sex and the erotic. For

Lorde, the erotic is a much bigger concept than sex. The erotic may be the energy you feel when you are having a great conversation, eating a scrumptious meal, painting a bookshelf, or watching two people dance salsa. Lorde believes that the erotic lies in a deeply female and spiritual plane.[15] It includes women's ability to give birth to a child—from darkness and safety into the mother's warm breast and the land of risk. The erotic starts with birth and, not surprisingly, can often be experienced in death, too—the incredibly intimate and distilled moment of saying good-bye to each other, of being in silence with someone's last breath. We are capable of feeling such intimacy during these times—moments of profound connection at the level of the energetic body. This is the erotic resting and playing and being in the world—an energy, kinetic impulse, power among us.

So what does the erotic have to do with brahmacharya? People often try to make sexual intimacy between each other both more and less than it is. We make it more when we try to use sex as a substitute for real talking, listening, and intimacy. Sex can be easy in that way—you can jump past conflicts, confusion, and hurt into the land of sex while sidestepping real honesty with each other. On the other hand, sex can often be treated as less than it is, too. Hooking up with strangers, exposing yourself to unsafe situations, having sex with a long-term partner in a kind of rote, unthinking way—are all examples of treating sexuality as less than what it can be.

Practicing brahmacharya encourages us to honestly deal with our own sexual histories. It is sad to realize that we often can't authentically identify what is beautiful and extraordinary about sexuality without dealing with violence. Meanwhile, I keep hearing the wise voice of Buddhist scholar Jan Willis, who talks about how Westerners tend to take what they want from Buddhist principles and leave the rest—to believe in the concept of meditation but not practice it consistently, to believe in the concept of nonviolence but then support militarism. That makes me wonder about brahmacharya as well. Are those who interpret this yama as sexual moderation instead of impeccable sexual behavior or celibacy taking the easy way out?

In Alistair Shearer's translation of the Yoga Sutras, the scholar interprets brahmacharya as "moving into the Immensity" or "living with Reality." Shearer objects to interpreting the concept as celibacy, explaining: "True yoga is a natural process, and has no place for repression, whether of the ego, sex or anything else. Such an attitude of forced control is against life, and can only result in strain and tension in the name of some supposedly 'higher' ideal." Shearer sees brahmacharya as "a state of self-sufficient wholeness, an innocence that is its own ecstasy."[16] This interpretation is worth contemplating. Exploring brahmacharya can be a juicy form of self-study (svadhyaya). It certainly asks us to tap into the energetic body. Understanding our ethics around sexuality tells us much about who we are as people. In the meantime, I will keep singing the words to Sweet Honey in the Rock's song, smiling.

How Ganesha Got His Elephant Head

At a yoga training I attended in Bali, in the mornings some of us gathered in front of Ganesha, the elephant god, to meditate before the 6:30 class. This particular Ganesha is especially round and jovial in his expression, perhaps because his trunk whimsically twirls above his head, giving the appearance of a grand, happy smile. We brought him offerings—fresh bright-orange marigolds that looked spectacular on his pearl-white body, a blue string of stones around his throat chakra, mala beads that cascade from his outstretched hands, a string of tea lights outlining the base upon which he sits. On a purely physical plane, it might seem strange to be sitting next to a carved piece of concrete, pouring out wishes and dreams, worries and intentions, but perhaps the combination of the mythology about Ganesha and the awareness of so many people coming before us with similar worries and prayers called us in.

Ganesha got his wide-open elephant ears and trunk because his father, Shiva, had cut off his head when Ganesha was still a boy. His mother, Parvati, had asked her son to stand guard outside the house while she took a bath. But his father, who didn't recognize him, took out a sword and cut off his son's head, believing him to be an intruder. Parvati was traumatized and told Shiva he must do something to pay homage. So Shiva asked an elephant to sacrifice his upper body for Ganesha. That is how the boy became half elephant. In the process, Ganesha became a being able to remove obstacles.

The mantra that is often recited to Ganesha is *Om gam ganapataye namaha,* which asks Ganesha to remove every impediment in your life. The way that Ganesha does this work, however, is not by plowing straight through barriers. Rather, Ganesha works around them. He may not help you pass your chemistry test but may show you that you love Spanish literature. He may not fix your relationship but may bring new love into your life. Ganesha knows that often the best way to win a battle is to not show up on the battlefield. Indeed, his father's violence is why he lost his head to begin with. Rather, Ganesha helps you find other ways of overcoming obstacles. Ultimately, he shows you how to tap into your own creativity to recognize new solutions.

This is what long-term yoga can bring to people—ways to find answers that don't demand a fight, that don't draw blood. Long-term yoga brings us new ways of handling conflict. This may come from being so physically stretched, sometimes psychically relaxed, that you don't have the energy to fight—it just feels too demanding. There is something about practicing lotus pose, extended hand to foot pose II, headstand cycle, full splits, and side crow (to name a few intense poses) that can squeeze conflict right out of you. Learning to walk away from strife may come from practicing, over and over again, how to come down silently on the mat, from down dog pose to lunge, from down dog to warrior one, from down dog to standing. Stepping softly from one place on the mat to another, using your core strength, coming from inside yourself rather than from outside, can become a way of being in the world as well—quiet, soft, from a strong base, not giving up your power needlessly but also being sturdy enough to be flexible when unexpected demands come in your direction. Learning to soften your gaze.

Moving through the world from a strong, soft place doesn't come all at once. Being able to draw wisdom from Ganesha doesn't come overnight, either. And these abilities are not easily measured. They don't announce themselves as a "ta-da" show stopper. They are subtle changes—in the ease of reclined butterfly pose *(supta baddha konasana)* or a slow slide into plow pose *(halasana)*. In the meantime, when I ask Ganesha for guidance, bringing an offering of another beautiful flower, one part of the mythology about Ganesha's origins still troubles me. How did the elephant feel about having to give up his head and ears and trunk for the son of Shiva and Parvati? Elephants have long memories, as is seen when they walk outside of their usual migratory path to visit the bones of their ancestors. They remember humans whom they bonded with decades before. Perhaps people who have been sacrificed—not only those who have lost their lives but those whose lives were in danger, who have had to walk through fire to save their own lives—may be those most likely to see Ganesha's origins from the elephant's point of view. If long-term yoga can help people see a dynamic from multiple perspectives simultaneously, that would include from the point of view of Shiva, Parvati, Ganesha, the ones praying to Ganesha, the elephant, *and* the elephant's kin.

May those praying to Ganesha learn to think creatively. May parents not cut off their children's heads. May those who sacrificed find regeneration. May some elephant somewhere take on whatever human body part might be helpful, perhaps the ability to walk upright, if the journey to her or his ancestors seems long.

Between Exhale and Inhale

> Taking refuge means committing your life to waking up, to taking on the problem of suffering and the end of suffering for all beings and ourselves. This is what zazen is about. Sitting upright in stillness means to see oneself in complete interdependence with all beings, with the rocks and trees and ocean and sky. The emptiness we so often talk about is not some kind of negative space. It is total interdependence.
>
> —Hozan Alan Senauke[17]

It wasn't until I had practiced yoga for years that I started to get some idea of the "emptiness" that Hozan Alan Senauke is talking about. For years, this whole concept completely eluded me. Twenty years ago I remember attending a lecture by meditation teacher Larry Rosenberg, where he talked about how what he most learned from his ten years of concentrated Zen meditation was "nothing." For several of those years he lived at an ashram, staring at a wall. I remember feeling stunned by this notion (actually feeling like I wanted to run out of the room when I heard it)—that he learned "nothing" from all that suffering. I didn't get it, that he was talking about a different "nothing" than I was thinking. For me, the idea of learning "nothing" was akin to losing time, having no proof of my existence, spinning in place, being stuck, lost, alone. Feeling that I am learning *something* everyday is how I have felt I am moving forward, that I can produce something meaningful, that I matter in the world.

Similarly, the commonly cited notion (in Buddhist and yoga circles) that our essence as human beings is emptiness has been baffling. Emptiness seemed like what I have been fighting against all of my life—the experience of not being able to find feelings inside of me, as if my chest were an empty cavern. It took me years in therapy to realize that the emptiness I felt was a consequence of having to abandon feelings a long time ago. And that a lot of my healing was connected to claiming those feelings again—as it turns out, one feeling at a time. So, in therapy in my twenties, my therapist and I "did" sadness for over a year. Then, for what seemed like a long time, I felt rage. Then, I started to find some nuance in my feelings—to be able to tell the difference between anger and frustration, sadness and loneliness, hunger and exhaustion. For me, healing started when I rediscovered feelings that I had lost touch with. So, I would have thought that healing was the opposite of feeling empty. Learning that my "self" was made up of feelings, that feelings lived in my body, was a crucial step away from emptiness. You can see why the idea of essence as emptiness would have been threatening, if not inconceivable, to me in my twenties. To think that who I am, at my core, is emptiness would have sounded like hell, being right back in the trauma where there were no feelings, nothing at all, just aloneness.

This is why it took me a long time to understand "emptiness" as a gracious feeling between exhale and inhale that I sometimes now feel. When the sky opens up and everything is calm. Emptiness (nothingness), a feeling of peace, of belonging, of connectedness to a calm collective consciousness. Emptiness—an experience of safety and openness. A blessed spot. For me, finding my feelings, one precious feeling at a time, was a way into finding breath. And breath was a way into "emptiness" and "nothingness" that I could look forward to, even seek out.

To Get Quiet

When my grandmother asked me to help her pass into another realm, a month shy of her 101st birthday, her instructions were clear. On the December day I arrived, the first thing she said to me was, "I need you to help me to go." Then, with a little pause, "I will miss you." And then, "Take care of yourself." After that, there were few lucid moments between us, although the intimacy born of decades of being bone close carried me. I called hospice, who, with a stunning array of soulful nurses, close relatives, and my chosen family, helped my grandmother discover a way out of the excruciating pain she was in so that she could find her way into another realm.

While the gifts of yoga have been many and varied, none has been more profound than how it prepared me to accompany my grandmother in her last two weeks. Because I was lucky enough to be with her around the clock, I could witness her journey, as the morphine started to relax her pain so the natural dying process could take over. During the day and especially at night I spent hours with her as I entered into a meditative space with her.[18] It was through her experience that I grasped, not just intellectually but somatically, why many yogis consider the sixth, seventh, and eighth limbs of yoga as interconnected. By finding a point of focus and concentration (dharana) on my own and my grandmother's breath, I was then able to find a flow in this concentration, which enabled me to do a meditation (dhyana) that connected me to her and to an expansive presence that she was entering into and that increasingly was all around her (samadhi).

What made me marvel was how being in tune with her breath gave me visual images that were guideposts on the journey. On the day before she passed, as I was meditating with her, I became aware of a golden bird that was stretching one of its wings and then lifted up into a gold space that was simultaneously a mountain, a cross, and a star. As I understood it, this was her process of dying, a sentient being (a bird) becoming (being absorbed into) a shape that was a combination of three powerful symbols. On the last full day of her living I became aware of energy in the shape of a globe that had beautiful burnt orange around its perimeter and was rising above her. While skeptics might say that these were in my imagination, my experience was that these energies or entities were right there with us in the unrestrained space that sometimes opens up during meditation.

Later that afternoon, when it appeared that my grandmother was just a few breaths from letting go, I was aware of her climbing up a waterfall the size of Niagara Falls, a reality that scared me because of the enormity of that task. Worse yet, when she had made it to the top of the waterfall fighting against an enormous current, there was a fast-moving reservoir of water, the texture of oil, gloppy, bubbling, menacing in its demeanor. I worried how she could possibly make her way through to safer space. An hour later, after having anticipated her passing, there was what felt like a hairpin turn in her process as a combination of bile and mucous came pouring out of her mouth. Her body changed from being relaxed and easy to extremely agitated and upright, as I and those around me worked hard to stem this process. In one of the only times in the previous two weeks, I found myself whispering words in her ear, trying to help her find belly breath since it seemed that her lungs had collapsed even as she was still breathing.[19] She did eventually start to breathe a little more easily, dropping into a space of breath that sounded like an original score of music—short, then fast; skipped beats and then long held breaths; whole, half, and quarter notes; staccato and then legato—until finally, a long pause and a final elegant, faint gasp, in the early morning hour of the second day of a new year.

In all of this I felt I was with her, my own breathing sometimes matching hers, sometimes quite different, but both of us in a spacious space somewhere together. In the minutes before her last breath, I saw sky, fast moving, bright-blue sky with little puffs of clouds zooming across the horizon. This is when I knew she would be okay, the climbing up a waterfall replaced by a whisking blue.

In those last days together, her slowing breath deepened mine as well as my ability to concentrate, to be in that meditative space with her, even when the static of medical beepers and walkie-talkies, distraught relatives, and flushing toilets threatened to steal me.[20] This is what Patanjali promises us in the Yoga Sutras: the slowing of the breath is interlinked with deep concentration.[21] This is what some moments with my gram required, that level of focus, to stay with her as she journeyed.

What a gift, though, when the single pointed focus of concentration opens up into meditation to help us find samadhi. In our last days together, I felt less that I was an individual person, her granddaughter, and more as if I were a collective presence, a representative from my family, a long lost lover, her mother, or a combination of all of them. In these moments, the intimacy in the air was so palpable that whether she knew "me" didn't seem relevant. As Charlotte Bell writes, "Samadhi happens when we let go of ourselves, our constructed identities, and merge with what is present."[22] This is what happened for me. I merged with what was present and could then accompany her as she went.

Now that my grandmother is off into another realm, I look for her in certain skies. I am finding her in my own breath, even in distractions that accompanied her last days. On the day before she slipped into a place where she could not communicate with me in words, I told her that even as she was dying she was being our teacher, the elder, this time teaching us about meditation. She, who had been meditating much of the time in the last several years of her life, in her chair, sometimes accompanied by Beethoven, sometimes by *Jane Eyre*, sometimes by an adoring relative. But mostly alone, teaching us to be there, quiet with her as well.

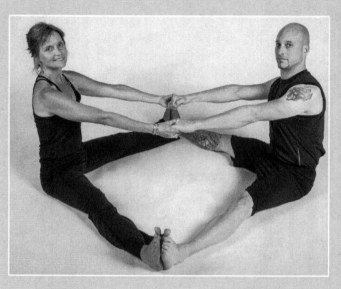

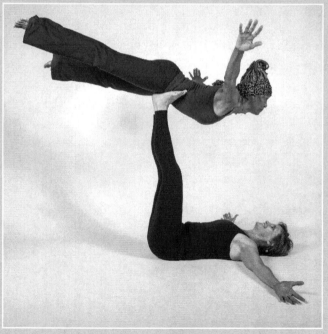

PART V

In the Shadow of the Temple

The Special Work of Teachers

The teacher who walks in the shadow of the temple, among his followers, gives not of his wisdom but rather of his faith and lovingness.

If he is indeed wise he does not bid you enter the house of his wisdom, but rather leads you to the threshold of your own mind.

—Kahlil Gibran[1]

Early in the Yoga Sutras, Patanjali identifies a number of experiences that can lead to the "threshold of your own mind"—becoming aware of inner radiance, inquiring about our dreams, and "being attuned to another mind that is itself unperturbed by desire."[2] Everybody deserves to be guided by mentors and teachers, people whose own minds have achieved the kind of freedom Patanjali refers to. But sometimes it is difficult for trauma survivors to ask for guidance. Survivor's guilt can get in the way of such seeking, and survivors wonder, "Why do I deserve experienced, wise teachers when others don't have them?" Or, "Who am I to ask for a teacher to give me attention, to really see me?" Sometimes survivors don't allow ourselves to want the guidance, or to acknowledge the need for it and think, "I have made it this far without a mentor, a teacher, so why would I want one now?"

We all deserve to be in the presence of those who have experienced moments of enlightenment, those whose yoga practice has brought them to a kinder, more whole place. Such presence can give us models for what is possible. In *The Heart of Yoga*, T. K. V. Desikachar, the son of Krishnamacharya, one of the best-known yogis of the modern era, writes, "When the Yoga Sutra was written it was taken for granted that students went to a teacher; that is why there is no specific reference to a teacher in the texts. Originally yoga was passed on by word of mouth; only much later was it written down. Students lived with their teachers until they got to know them well."[3] We all need teachers who will, with their humility, love of the practice, and zest for life, bring us to new awareness, teachers who choose to walk in the shadow of the temple, not right in front, knowing that the best teacher is the one who can find the teacher within the student.

Part of what excites me about yoga is realizing how yoga teachers can lead the way in creating healing spaces. Until recently few medical personnel, educators, social workers, and community activists received somatic training in how to work with trauma survivors. That's where yoga comes in. With its systematic methods for healing at the level of the body as well as the mind and spirit, it can offer invaluable help to those working with survivors. The enlightened yoga teacher is someone who has learned through yoga how to tap into all the levels of being, knows how to listen, how to sense through the body what the student needs, and then how to vary the practice according to those needs. This ability to adapt the practice to the individual is particularly crucial in interactions with trauma survivors. For some of us, getting hands-on assistance during a class is a way to feel seen, to be brought back into our bodies as the teacher's touch reminds us that we are here. For other people, however, assists can feel invasive, disruptive. And there are also those who once thrived on assists but are now going through a period of wanting no touch at all.

As the teacher, being in the moment and staying attentive to one's students are crucial, as is recognizing that they are the ultimate experts in what they need. But having said that, it is necessary to acknowledge that teachers can't do the right thing all the time. At a weekend training, the pioneering brain researcher and trauma expert Bessel A. van der Kolk talked about how those of us who work with trauma survivors will inevitably make mistakes when it comes to trying to respect boundaries.[4] This is true no matter how much we study, how much we know, or how well-intentioned we are. So we must start and end this work from a place of humility. Staying nondefensive is essential, as is flexibility. Cookie-cutter yoga isn't sufficient when it comes to survivors.

Good teachers come in all kinds of packages, including some surprising ones, as is described below in "The Fire-Fighting Yoga Instructor" and "All of Us in This World." Among the most gifted teachers are those who both work with trauma and are survivors themselves—a combination that takes guts in a culture that still asks healers to hide our lived experience in the name of professionalism. Ultimately, experience also teaches us that some of the most profound teachers are not the ones in front of the class. They are the ones on the mat right next to us, as comes out in "Multiplying Joy." The search is worth it. Definitely.

The Fire-Fighting Yoga Instructor

In some of the instruction material for yoga teachers whose practice is geared toward trauma survivors, I have often seen the suggestion that teachers use a soothing voice when we speak—that talking in a calm, slow voice can model for students a similar attitude and approach. A peaceful, carefully modulated voice does encourage an atmosphere in which students don't feel rushed, or pushed to perform, or uncomfortable about allowing their feelings to surface.

At the same time, I have to admit that one of my all-time favorite yoga instructors (from whom I have taken classes regularly over the last decade) is an ex-fireman, vet, and union organizer who teaches as if his students need to be saved from a fire—barking instructions, shouting at us to tighten our quads, suck in our stomachs, and not be afraid to "make it hurt," getting ever more urgent in tone and intensity as the class progresses. Ron is someone who will come over and rest all 180 pounds of himself on my shins when I am on my back, knees pulled to my chest in wind removing pose (pavanamuktasana), reminding me to "breathe" (who is he kidding?). If he sees people looking a little dazed and dizzy after coming up from camel pose (ustrasana), he's been known to say, "Enjoy that feeling; it's a lot like living in the sixties again." He also says things like, "This next posture is a bitch of a pose," and, "This is the pose I hate the most in the sequence, and always have." He often tells the class that it took him years to be able to do certain poses, and just as often advises us not to worry about whether we can do all of the poses correctly since we might need at least this lifetime and perhaps another to master them.

But I keep going back to Ron's class. Many others keep going back, too, because when Ron is leading the class, we know we are in the hands of a consummate teacher. For me, far more important than whether teachers have calm voices is how authentic they are—how much of their true selves they allow into their teaching. So, while many survivors may prefer soothing voices, I would say that just as important is what is delicately referred to as the "bullshit factor." Survivors seem to be especially wary of people who are not themselves, who try to affect a sweetness or calm that they don't in fact possess. Ron, on the other hand, in all his bluster and bravado, is one of the most real people I have ever met—vociferous in his condemnation of duplicitous politicians, stalwart in his support of racial equity, and forthright in his critique of Bikram's numerous fancy cars.[5] In his booming voice, Ron will command us in French, English, and Sanskrit, informing us that we didn't get up early to act like wimps, sometimes shouting so much that he makes himself hoarse. And with his six-foot, three-inch frame, he will crawl on the floor next to a newcomer to be sure her heels are in alignment as she tucks her head to her knees in rabbit pose *(sasangasana)*. Or he'll stay late to help someone with a pose that isn't in the official series. He does all this while ostensibly teaching a style of yoga where hands-on assists are frowned upon, where teachers are required, even policed, to stick with the scripted dialogue.

Several years ago, to celebrate his sixtieth birthday, Ron took sixty Bikram classes in sixty days. No small feat. Week after week, Ron pushes us the same way he pushed himself during those two months. He tells us "never give up on yourselves," and we don't, because we know he has given us everything he has.

Fierce Is a Quality of Light

> Now I understand that some of my gifts are to induce cataclysm
> and to be a Truth Speaker—someone who is committed to speak-
> ing about difficult and hidden things, to revealing the beauty in the
> world in order to teach and heal.
> —Ana T. Forrest[6]

While it makes sense that many people who become yoga teachers are also trauma survivors, few speak openly about this. There is still a fissure between being a professional and sharing your own story, an unspoken taboo about such a disclosure—as if such telling will detract from your own skills and insights. Several years ago, when I was delivering a key-note lecture at a national eating disorders conference (along with Bessel A. van der Kolk), I prefaced my talk by saying that in addition to being a sociologist and ethnographer, I also came as someone healing from an eating problem, that this experience had helped in my research. In the evaluations I received a few weeks later, several people in the audience commented that my self-disclosure was "unprofessional" and had made my talk suspect in their eyes.

The pressure to censor our own vulnerabilities and expertise makes Ana T. Forrest's memoir about her work as a teacher and visionary both unique and brave. In *Fierce Medicine* she is not only explicit about traumas that she faced (childhood physical, emotional, and sexual abuse) and ways she coped (bulimia, alcoholism, suicide attempts); she also gives us insight about how the trauma informs her own teaching. One of the signature techniques in Forrest's approach is that people breathe into an area of their body that is tweaky or injured, sending breath and attention to that spot. Forrest's incorporation of this helpful tool came partly from her learning to do this herself as she was healing, discovering that such concentration (dharana) can bring insight about what that area is saying—how it might be storing information (and memory) that needs to be released. Forrest writes, "Our bodies tell our stories, and they always tell the truth when we listen. I want to help you hear your body's story, and then teach it to speak its truth."[7]

Another teaching that is unique to Forrest's approach is her abdominal work—an exacting, intense series of cues that inevitably let you know you have a core that runs deep inside of you. This core work, in addition to building the physical stamina that is key to supporting most all of the postures, also helps people find that part of themselves. During the years when she was bingeing and bulimic, Forrest remembers "my stomach hurt, but only from a dull distance, as if it didn't belong to me."[8] She also understands how sexual abuse shuts down a woman's connection to her abdomen and pelvis. Forrest's own willingness to become attached and respectful to her core gave her the wisdom to design core-enlivening techniques to help others as well. She asks of us, "If you can restore that core fire, that magma, that heartbeat of the earth, what would be ignited in your creativity, your cell structure, your body's ability to cleanse and renew itself? This is a very primal place: life, sex, security, procreation, species survival, shelter. It's where the flames of the life force are."[9]

You can also tell that Forrest's yoga was made possible from her own trauma history because she takes no prisoners. There is a reason that the title of her book is *Fierce Medicine.*[10] She detoxed from alcohol, cigarettes, and drugs during her first yoga teacher training at eighteen years old. She sat through classes on Buddha and Patanjali while hallucinating from drug withdrawal. She did dozens of sun salutations (surya namaskar) in a row each night. Her focus on this ancient and graceful series of standing, bowing, and stretching poses that are linked with the breath were her step away from the habit and familiarity of addiction. Forrest knows that yoga can save your life because it saved hers and that you have to be disciplined to receive its healing. She defines dharma as "what you do with what has been done to you."[11]

For Forrest, such determination has meant opening herself to the wisdom of many other teachers. She has also walked away from teachers whose egos, rigidity, or exploitation stood in the way of her own practice. Once she realized he was exploiting her, Forrest walked out of a relationship with a lover whom she had written a yoga book with, had traveled and taught with all over the world. She even said good-bye to B. K. S. Iyengar, one of the most revered yogis in the world, after she felt he was trying to control her ingenuity and individuality.[12] And, in her teaching, she has stared several orthodoxies in the face, including the belief that the ultimate goal is to transcend, rather than fully inhabit, the body.

Such a willingness to question a party line speaks to Forrest's own multilayered journey, including her lessons from living by the Columbia River in Washington State under the tutelage of a Cherokee medicine man, Heyoka. From him and other Native American healers, Forrest learned to call in the energy and protective power of the Four Directions, a ritual she performs to ready a space before teaching. People who have taken her workshops and classes know the power emanating from a studio that Forrest has blessed. Forrest seems cognizant of the damage of white shamanism—white stealing of Native American rituals, knowledge, and expertise—while devoted to honoring and drawing upon the energy of the land she teaches on in the United States (all of which was originally Native American land).[13] She sees her work as "Mending the Hoop of the People," a calling that recognizes a range of traumas that includes the attempted genocide of Indigenous people.[14] Her grounding in the earth and use of ritual teaches us that healing the body and the land go together. She writes, "When you walk the red road . . . you're aware of the energy around you. You're open to the Beauty in the world and choose to consciously embody Beauty as you move through life."[15] From Ana T. Forrest we see that environmental justice, including the recognition of Indigenous sovereignty, becomes the eagle pose (garudasana) for yoga-in-action.

The Chickpea and the Pot

One of the common characteristics among trauma survivors who are also yoga teachers is their willingness to draw upon a wide range of sources to create innovative teaching methods. This creativity may partly come from the reality that there isn't much out there yet about how to teach yoga *as* survivors. Survivors who are also yoga instructors are carving an image in the void as our own teaching evolves. It is also true that our eclectic, kitchen-sink teaching methods parallel how survivors heal ourselves; the journey that often looks like patchwork is, itself, a creative process.

The teaching methods that trauma survivors develop are beautifully exemplified by Max, a professor of religion at Vassar College who has been teaching yoga for fifteen years. Max has struggled with depression intermittently since she was fourteen, including devastating bouts immediately following an abortion, after the birth of her daughter, and in the wake of a painful divorce. She was in a near-fatal car crash and has had several serious surgeries, and two of her brother's roommates were killed in the 9/11 attacks. She also somehow made it through years of graduate school and early years as a professor with a serious undiagnosed case of ADHD. Through all this, yoga has been a mainstay, a reality that led her to teach yoga even as she is also a single mother, an untenured professor, and a scholar of Sufi mysticism and comparative religions.

As a yoga teacher, Max has learned to bring her whole self to the practice even as her early precise Iyengar-based training (and her own skepticism about yoga's spiritual dimensions) made little room for the pastiche teaching style she eventually developed. She opens her classes with often hilarious, seriously original, dharma talks that draw upon her research. One of her classic dharma stories involves a Rumi poem, "Chickpea to Cook," wherein a chickpea first protests boiling in a pot as a cook swats it back into the water. Finally, the chickpea burns into a new state, free of its old container, experiencing ecstasy in its new form. This chickpea's transformation, Max proclaims, can teach us about the fire of purification (*tapas,* the third niyama) about how yoga (and life) require focused energy, discipline, and the burning away of old patterns. In other dharma talk, Max speaks about purity and simplicity (sauca, the first niyama), commenting on Iyengar's recommendation that yoga teachers bookend their teaching with hot showers, first to purify themselves before teaching and then to release old energy gathered during the practice. This yoga absolution closely approximates Muslim purification ceremonies, the attention to the Sabbath in Judaism, and early Protestant attention to cleanliness and order.

This attention to the spiritual dimensions of Max's teaching didn't come easily. In fact, for the first several years, the physical postures were all she was interested in. She loved seeing what her body could do—flipping into handstands, figuring out how to do deep backbends, finding the edge of her flexibility and then extending it. But then, after walking away from a car crash in which the car was almost completely flattened, she found the sandalwood beads that had been hanging on the mirror bursting with a scent that had left them years before. She had bought the beads outside of a shrine of a long dead Sufi devotee who was miraculously healed after suffering paralysis from an accident. After interpreting the sandalwood beads and her inexplicable survival from the car crash as a sign, Max began considering a realm in yoga beyond the intellect, a realm found through life experience, sometimes amid trauma. This journey enables Max to reach out as a teacher to those most focused on the physical as well as those craving a spiritual connection—to understand students' resistance to what Max considers the religious aspects of yoga, as well as their potential hunger for it.[16]

Max's experiences with trauma also make her a believer in working within community, of expanding the network of healers around her. Just as consciousness can expand with practice, Max makes it her business to see that the healers she knows include psychotherapists, physical therapists, energy workers, nutritionists, herbalists, psychics, physicians, and intellectuals so that she can best help her students. From Max's perspective, it is not enough to say, "You might want to seek out a therapist," or "What does your doctor say about your hip pain?" While her official training as a yoga teacher emphasized her focus on the asanas and breath work, as a survivor she came to see it as her responsibility to offer people specific referrals and resources beyond yoga to find the healing they need. This, too, came from her own experience as someone who spent years unsuccessfully trying to use yoga to fix symptoms she later came to understand as ADHD. It was only after an official diagnosis by a trained health professional and proper medication that she saw real change. From this and other experiences, Max saw that yoga can't be the end-all, be-all for people, especially for survivors.

Max's willingness to think out of the box also extends to her eclectic teaching style that combines what she describes as her "take charge military approach" with playful and scrappy improvisations. She knows from experience that the last thing that trauma survivors need is a pity party. They need to know they can do a whole lot more than they thought they could, the sooner the better. That is why Max has been known to help people up into headstands very early in their practice, sometimes their first session, which she believes builds confidence. She also makes sure that, even when her classes are packed, she gives everyone a neck rub with oil at the end of class while they are in savasana.

Even as she does this, Max is reticent to call herself a healer, a word that seems too big and evolved for how she feels. Instead, she reasons that if she keeps acting like a healer, someday she might actually become one, based on an adage she lives by—"If you keep doing something, it will eventually do you." While she is always a wry skeptic of her own abilities, people consistently tell her that the neck rub is the single most important motivation for coming to practice. In this way, I suspect that she, and many other trauma survivor teachers, go against the orthodoxy in many yoga circles, that yoga instructors avoid touch because it might restimulate trauma. For Max, the possibility of restimulating isolation and aloneness is far riskier than touch based on the intention to heal.

"The Issues Live in Our Tissues"

For yoga teachers who are trauma survivors themselves, creating classes that speak to lessons they have learned takes persistence. In the case of Kyczy Hawk, a yoga teacher and potter living in California, such willingness began with wanting to fuse the spiritual dimensions of twelve-step recovery programs with the physical health that yoga promises. As a recovering alcoholic, Hawk discovered that while Alcoholics Anonymous helped her stop drinking and become part of a community of people recovering from addictions, she was still yearning for help with physical healing (poor eating, joint pain, shallow breathing, lack of physical stamina). As she practiced yoga herself, she began to see a deep resonance between the spiritual dimensions of yoga (including the yamas and niyamas) and the twelve steps.

This is when Hawk got busy. In addition to linking up with the growing community of people who see how twelve-step recovery programs and yoga can be interwoven, she wrote *Yoga and the Twelve-Step Path*. In this book she teaches us that while addiction to alcohol, food, and drugs has a physiological basis, the roots of these addictions often stem from trauma. As someone who was raised by an actively alcoholic mother and an angry and disengaged father, Hawk learned early how to be the family's caretaker. By ninth grade, she was smoking pot and taking diet pills; drinking wine and doing drugs followed. Soon a split developed between the good girl (managing the house, her studies) and the bad girl (reckless, truant at school, depressed). This split worsened through college and early years as a parent until she sought help. Her road to recovery was not smooth, but did, over time, bring her long-term abstinence and a steady yoga practice.

Hawk found that combining a twelve-step recovery with the eight limbs of yoga helps people see how addictions often begin as ways of coping. The compassion for self at the base of both practices has a way of welcoming people into studios and meeting halls, a reality that led Hawk to see why she is drawn to yoga classes that are structured like meetings—where people have a chance to say their names, are reminded that they are accepted as they are, and are supported in sharing their stories with others. Isolation and shame are two common dimensions for both trauma survivors and addicts. This is why yoga classes that specifically counter isolation by fostering community can be so helpful.

Hawk's own journey also helped her recognize how physical and emotional releases go hand in hand. This lesson came early in her yoga practice. One day, when she was feeling stiff and achy while attempting a seated forward fold (paschimottanasana), her teacher told the class that they had stamina stored in their bodies just waiting to be discovered. At that point, Hawk "burst into tears as something in my hips let go, and I realized that I could be strong without being isolated; I could stand on my own two feet while being taught, and I did not need to go it alone. What a concept! I have no idea where the thoughts or the tears came from. All I know is that there was tightness and resistance one moment, and softness and acceptance the next. Yoga practice forged the path for this moment of integration."[17]

Hawk's experience also taught her the value of classes where students are encouraged to take it easy. Teachers who incorporate modifications with props and adjustments in poses take into account that trauma trapped in people's muscles can register as physical pain. As Nikki Myers, a yoga therapist who designed the path-breaking yoga and twelve-step recovery program Y12SR has wisely said, "the issues live in our tissues."[18] This reality means that trauma-sensitive teaching pays close attention to the breath, since, as Hawk explains to her students, "the breath will never lie." If the breath is halting or jagged or stops entirely, these are clues that people are overdoing it. As Hawk writes, "Be kind; let the feelings come and let them go. Release the tension and come back into the pose with kindness. The intention of bringing body, mind, and spirit together is harmony."[19]

Dissociation on the Mat

During my first yoga teacher training, six months into the weekend sessions, the lead teacher announced that we would start the day with practicing Thai massage with a partner for two hours. I hadn't expected to do massage training that day, especially that early, and so had not done whatever psychic steeling of myself I do before people I barely know start to work their hands over my body. The instructions were to go into pigeon pose (eka pada raja kapotasana) and stay there for an extended period while the person practicing the massage would press down on our lower backs to extend the stretch. My body was already creaky and aching. That worried me. I couldn't understand why pigeon was feeling so awful, and I was getting more upset as the pose continued to be painful. In the moment, I didn't know how to come out of the pose without admitting defeat and that something was wrong.

Lucky for me, the woman who was practicing the massage technique on my body started to notice that something wasn't right—that I wasn't breathing, at all. By then, it was too late, though, I was already dissociating, scattering around the room, pieces of me on the wall like a pumpkin kids throw on Halloween. Feeling invisible, empty, missing, vague, gone. I had a sense of being in the room and not at the same time. My legs and arms felt there, but not there, huge in size, bloated like a snowman, prickly, like water turning into flotsam, floating and sinking. I began thinking, "I have to get out of here, escape without anyone noticing." After what seemed like a long time (what must have been just minutes), I was able to pull myself up from the pose and excuse myself, fleeing the room.

I don't remember leaving, but I recall being outside in the hall, starting to think that if I could just get to my phone and dial friends' numbers, and let them hear my voice, then maybe . . . I am not sure what exactly . . . but I had this desperate feeling of needing to call as soon as possible. All I could think was, look for a room, a hiding space, a place where I could make a call. I became vaguely aware that the woman who had been my massage partner was asking me if I was okay, my eyes darting, asking me if she could stay with me. While I didn't want to be rude, I couldn't understand why she didn't somehow simply know I needed to call people who love me right away? At that point I felt desperate. I knew my splintering wasn't her fault but I also didn't want to worry about her feelings either. Another voice was saying, she was being quiet and had found us a soft place, so maybe I could postpone calling my friends. I tucked my phone away so she couldn't see it.

I began to tell her in fragmented phrases that I dissociated and that, in the rare instances when this still happens, it typically takes fifteen to twenty minutes for me to come back together. I told her that I didn't want to do it too fast, because the process can be so jarring and jagged. She seemed fine about just sitting like a protective lion. We started talking in half sentences; more than that felt too overwhelming. The room started to feel like it had four walls, with a couch, a rug, with incense coming from the massage room next door. Smell was beginning to work again. I stood up, my limbs feeling a little bit like the skeleton we had studied the day before—attached but not. Together, but in pieces. Eventually when I returned to the classroom, I realized that the lead teacher, who was stretched with group dynamics in the room, hadn't noticed I had slipped out; and that I had been lucky that my classmate had followed me when I had left.

Later that day, I watched my hand go up, my mouth saying that I would like to facilitate a session on working with trauma survivors. I didn't use the first person, but I am guessing that there was something in my voice that revealed my experience. The lead teacher agreed. People seemed amenable. The woman who had accompanied me turned to me and whispered that it shouldn't be on me to be the educator. I smiled, grateful for her wisdom. Later, she sent me a beautiful essay about a time when she dissociated in class. I started to realize that I didn't need to facilitate the session alone. She would be there too with her many years as a therapist as welcome company. She offered to make a talking stick so that people could have something powerful and wise to hold when they talked about their own experience as teachers, their own experience with trauma.

As we planned the session, she told me what it was like to be next to me when I started to split into parts and then disappear. "Your whole body was armor, like a perfectly appointed car, maybe a Lexus. There was no air getting in or out. In fact, it seemed like you had stopped breathing entirely. I am not sure I have ever witnessed anyone being able to go that long without a breath." I smiled at her awareness, what it means to excel at surviving without breath for long periods of time. In a poem I wrote many years ago titled "You Know Survivors, We," the last line reads, "asphyxiation, a common calamity we tender."[20] Jokingly, I asked her if my body really felt like a Lexus. The image I had was of an Oldsmobile in Cuba, one of those very old cars that people have managed to keep on the road for decades, since the U.S. embargo has made getting new cars into Cuba nearly impossible. She tells me that I was definitely a Lexus; the old Cuban cars are much too drafty considering that I was sealed shut. We laughed at the imagery—car talk to describe human bodies when safety has momentarily disappeared.

The day of the workshop, we arrived with the gorgeous talking stick to brave and tender sharing from the teachers-in-training. What began as two of us wanting to talk about teaching and trauma became a collective process where everyone took risks. Some people spoke a lot. Others were quiet. But everyone, including the lead teacher, took risks by showing up and listening. People talked about eating problems, divorce, childhood loss, sexual abuse, and addictions. What was planned to be a one-hour session became much longer as people moved in closer to each other, a quiet collective presence forming around us. We talked about how working with survivors needs to start with having compassion for our own struggles. And how we can be a witnessing presence for ourselves and our students by honoring resilience and honesty.[21] While students may be hesitant to name their traumas, if we model this in sensitive and thoughtful ways, more space will open up for people to practice with ease. This became a project all of us can take up, a collective endeavor, a necessary part of becoming healing teachers.

It's All Brave

Sometimes, what has most struck me as a teacher, actually moved me to tears of gratitude and awe, has been the courage that people are willing to show when they first come to the mat. I am thinking, for example, of a woman who, after years of thinking about trying yoga, came to one of my classes. At the end, when I asked people how they were doing—and for reflections about the class—she said that when I suggested that people close their eyes during savasana, she actually did. Afterward, she told the group that for the first time in her life she was willing to close her eyes even though there were people around her—before, she had always been afraid that something "bad" might happen if her eyes were closed. A few of the women around her nodded in recognition of her spoken fear. I was reminded again about what it takes for so many people to feel safe in the world—the kind of alertness that we practice—often without even knowing it, to try to keep ourselves and those around us protected.

I am thinking too of the woman who speaks Urdu and very little English, who kept coming back even though her only real cues for how to do the postures came from what she saw modeled around her. She practiced with a headscarf, socks, long pants, and a big smile. Embarrassingly, I had to ask her name three times before I was able to pronounce it correctly. At first when she stretched out on her mat in the most comfortable position she could find, her head was cranked far to the left and straightening her legs didn't feel right to her at all. Still she kept coming back.

I am also thinking about a time I was teaching a class at a conference when, at the end of a meditation, everyone opened their eyes except for one woman in her forties, who was deep inside herself. When I noticed people's eyes on her (she was to my immediate left and so only in my peripheral vision), I looked over to see that she was sucking her thumb. A couple of the women started to laugh, probably uncomfortable with her gesture. I jumped in as soon as I could, making reference to how, during the meditation, I had been overwhelmed by how beautiful the people were in the circle. My silent wish was for a blanket of loving acceptance around this woman's body, an awareness on her part that the human body remembers what is comforting and returns to it—that this doubling back is healthy, makes sense. She slipped out early, as I tried to find her eyes, to try to tell her I hoped she would return to yoga.

It is brave to show up, even if it is with socks on for one month, six months, a year and counting. It is brave to close your eyes. It is brave to go inside enough to remember one's body in a time before injury intervened. It's all brave.

Multiplying Joy

Although I love going to yoga classes, I know there are great benefits to having a home practice as well. First, if you are ever stranded some-where—at an airport, on the highway when your car breaks down—if you have your mat with you, you can roll it out and do your practice wherever you are. A home practice also makes it easy to hear your own breath. Over the years, I have seen people really claim their practice after doing it alone for an extended period. They make it more definitively their own; they enter into poses more deeply and are more present in their bodies. A home practice is also essential when you are learning sequences by heart. It is one thing to do the poses on the cues of a terrific teacher; it is something else to be able to offer succinct and clear cues yourself. That takes practice, some of which you may do with others in the room, but much of which you have to do alone, talking your way through instruc-tions for the poses until they become a part of you.

There are many positive things to be said about a home practice. But there are at least as many reasons for complementing your home prac-tice with finding a studio with good teachers and fellow students whose company inspires you. For many of us, being able to practice the pos-tures while someone else is talking can help us give ourselves over to the practice more completely. My first yoga teacher, the remarkable Diane Ducharme, sometimes used the expression—"my brain, your body." Doing your practice to someone else's cues allows you to turn down your mental chatter a bit—to get into the zone as you ride the instructor's voice and just let it take you through your poses. Often it is easier to listen to your body if you don't have to think at the same time. All you have to do is follow the cues and move to the rhythm of your breath.

I also appreciate practicing with others because it can give you a con-tagious dose of prana. Have you ever noticed that when people are doing exactly what they are meant to do in the world, are right in the center of their passion, dropping down into a standing pose and then staying there perfectly balanced—that everyone around them is magnetized to that action? Prana is like a magnet; it draws you in. And prana is infectious. If people around you are feeling it, it can help you feel it, too. Prana can be collectively produced—the more people there are to generate the prana, the more of it there is, and the more likely it is that others will keep joining in. Prana is electric; it wires us all together. Prana is like an energetic form of serotonin, a natural caffeine. Everybody could use exposure to this "drug," perhaps trauma survivors especially, because prana carries hope. Prana makes you smile, makes you feel alive, leads you to dwell in the land of possibility.

Another reason I encourage studio practice is that sometimes you meet people there whom you would miss if you were at home, and one of those people might be just the person you need to know at this moment in your life. Why? Because often the most profound teachers aren't the ones standing at the front of the class, guiding students through the postures, but your fellow mat huggers. Who knows who might settle down on a mat next to you? The person destined to be your future partner? Someone who wrote the book you have been raving about for the last month? Or a vibrantly healthy woman who just passed the five-year survival mark after treatment for breast cancer, while you or someone you love has just been diagnosed with the disease? The connections you make through yoga so often turn out to be fortuitous, perhaps because it draws like-minded people together in such an intimate way, sweating together on their mats, falling out of side by side crow poses (bakasana), wobbling back and forth in tree (vrksasana).

As a practice that encourages people to turn upside down for extended periods, to lie on their backs and pretend they are dead bugs, to contort themselves into binds that seem to defy human anatomy, yoga gives us a chance to see each other in new and unexpected ways—and to laugh at ourselves. That is good for everyone, perhaps most especially for those who have gone through too much in their lives, who can benefit from being with others who are also going about the business of multiplying joy. For those struggling with isolation and loneliness, going to the studio helps counter these feelings, one yoga practice at a time.

From This One Woman's Body

I recently came back from a yoga retreat that was led by a well-known yoga teacher and author whom I have long respected. During his lectures he offered pithy and thoughtful analysis on yoga philosophy while making room for people's confusions and questions. He taught the asana portion of the weekend with passion—leading us through some of the most peaceful and grounded flows I have experienced. And around the edges—before and after classes—he brought palpable attentiveness to his interactions. As someone who has participated in his weekend retreats before, I found myself grateful again—that he has committed his life to yoga, that he has the dual gifts of writing and teaching, and that he knows how to brilliantly connect the subject of his lectures with the lessons underlying his asana practice.

At the same time, as the weekend progressed I found myself feeling tight in my shoulders, tight behind my eyes, sometimes a sign that I am carrying something I don't yet have words for, haven't yet faced. Thinking back over the weekend I wondered why this teacher, as honorable and knowledgeable as he is, didn't seem to know ways that he was sidestepping an awareness of trauma. For example, on the first night of the workshop, during the yoga practice, the second asana he included was happy baby, a pose that requires opening of the hips while exposing the groin area to the sky. It is not that this pose should be off limits, but to do it so early in the class, before we have gotten fully into our breaths and are aware of what feels safe, can be risky.

Early in the class, he also asked us to turn to a partner and help to open her or his meridians by patting down their shoulders, arms, back, back of the legs, and feet. We hadn't even learned each other's names in this retreat yet. I found myself darting my eyes around, seeing whom I could most comfortably partner with among the strangers. I then realized that I needed to go to the back of the room if I was going to attempt to do this exercise, away from people's gazes. So, I found myself needing to explain to the perfect stranger I had partnered up with that I felt better being at the back of the class, and then trying to relax as this woman started patting me down from behind. As she did, I kept thinking about people who have been patted down for real—at airports, on the streets, among communities where frisking is disproportionately practiced.

And I thought about how, even though I am a feminist and have been writing about and thinking about trauma for years, I didn't have whatever courage or energy I needed to speak up and say that I didn't feel comfortable patting down a stranger or being patted down myself, that happy baby early in the sequence was too much, that a teacher's soothing voice without knowledge is not enough.

Today's prayer, for me, is a question: What will it take for trauma survivors ourselves to be at the center of classes, trainings, and workshops where issues of trauma arise? If, as the poet and activist June Jordan wrote, "we are the ones we are waiting for,"[22] then what will it take for us to know that we have arrived?

In *The Heart of Yoga*, Desikachar writes that the qualities of relaxation and gentleness *(sukha)* and strength and steadiness *(sthira)* can be envisioned through the Indian mythology of Ananta, the king of snakes. Ananta's body is soft and gentle enough (sukha) and firm and steady enough (sthira) to "support the universe."[23] Today, my feeling is that we will need all of these qualities to remember what we know, to speak about what we think and feel, to know that justice begins with our bodies.

Families of Canaries

> It's always possible that the teacher leading the class may not be
> ready. A possible problem arises when the yoga instructor, out of
> fear or inexperience, or even a misguided caring for the student,
> seeks to limit the student's experience. In so doing, the situation
> may duplicate the original traumatic experience in which the stu-
> dent may have felt unheard or even shamed.
> —Amy Weintraub[24]

It's hard when the very teacher we seek for healing causes hurt, shame, or
confusion. The truth is that while there has been increasing attention to
what trauma-sensitive yoga might look like, many yoga teachers haven't
yet had the experience and training that might make this reality. Kripalu,
the oldest and largest yoga retreat in the United States, recently initiated a
landmark study on yoga and veterans with PTSD.[25] The Trauma Center,
in Brookline, Massachusetts, has a program that teaches yoga instructors specific techniques for working with trauma survivors. All over the
country, there are grassroots programs where people who are incarcerated
practice yoga to counter the assaults on the human spirit they experience
daily in prison.

While these projects are leading the way in developing pedagogies
that are trauma sensitive, many yoga students end up stumbling through
a number of yoga teachers until they find someone who "gets it." In the
meantime, it is easy to think we are being too demanding, that we should
just get over it, that yoga instructors shouldn't be expected to deal with
trauma. These are the voices to quiet, the ones that ask us to suck it up
and move on. Being careful about how assists are done, including asking
permission before touching someone, is good policy for everyone. Making time and space for people to talk about how their practice shaped
how they are feeling emotionally is good for everyone. As canaries in a
yoga practice, we need to keep chirping, as regularly as we can, in pairs,
triads, and entire extended aviary families, if that is what it takes. Amy
Weintraub writes, "It's important that you find a teacher you trust and a

class where you feel safe. Psychologists call this a 'holding environment.' It's the place we feel safe enough to do emotional work. In the context of a yoga class, you want to be free enough to do emotional work. . . . You want to be free to experience what is most authentic about yourself, without the risk of feeling judged."[26]

Like Jazz

[In jazz] there's the importance of developing and finding your own perspective and having pride in yourself. That's what we call a solo. Swing is about learning how to negotiate and how to be flexible. Then there's improvisation, which teaches us to use our intelligence and all the things at our disposal to respond appropriately to the moment at hand. The Blues recognizes tragedy, but always with optimism. Things might be tragic, but they are going to get better. Optimism that is not naïve in the face of adversity—something is wrong, but we're going to make it better.
—Wynton Marsalis[27]

At a recent, end-of-the-year yoga class, I planned to guide people through a sequence that centered on triangle pose *(trikonasana)*, one of the sturdiest of shapes, the three legs of a stool capable of keeping a seat balanced under formidable weight. It made sense to end the year with this pose and others that stand around it—side plank *(vasisthasana)*, revolved extended side angle *(parivrtta parsvakonasana)*, and prayer twist *(parivrtta utkatasana)*. Only on this particular day, after doing some flowing sun salutations together, one of the women announced that we should dance instead. "Remember," she said, "a few months ago when we did that circle thing, all of us threading through each other? We need to dance today."

I must have looked at her with such a whimsical expression, this suggestion coming from a woman in her sixties who had been known to mutter under her breath in relation to most poses, who often comes in late shaking her head and sometimes leaves shaking her head, too, whose Caribbean upbringing signals formality—a reserved and proper way of dealing with people. This is a woman who, when I asked people to introduce themselves and share one celebration about their bodies, consistently said, "Well, I got up this morning. That's enough."

So, at her insistence, we danced to Chaka Khan, Stevie Wonder, and Van Morrison, our bodies ribboning through each other, wrapping and unwrapping like an elaborate Möbius strip. I am not sure why, but I made a suggestion it might be good to end the year with headstands. When I asked if they were up for that, there was total silence in the room, until the woman who first requested the dancing says, "Well, if we gotta do it, we might as well get started."

Now, I should say that a few of them had never done headstands (at least as adults). But with assistance, all of them were able to fling their legs up in the air in tripod headstand, the others cheering them on, all of them in shock as they came down. Delight in the air had transformed itself into a kind of awe, their energy making me giddy, leading me to say, "let's do legs up the wall pose, let's *viparita karani* our way into the new year." Only when we got there, one of the students started talking about how she had been watching a show on yoga on TV when she saw someone do this "upside down thing and then walk across the room." Piecing her description together, I guessed she was talking about wheel (urdhva dhanurasana), which I then flipped into, saying that in the new year, we could start working toward such a posture. Only the woman who had initiated the dance had begun figuring out how to do it herself. I jumped up from my upside-down pose, saying I had to watch her every second for fear that she might do something crazy as she started to hike herself up, everyone else laughing, delighting in her ingenuity, their butts against the walls, legs toward the sky.

Another student said that he felt so high it reminded him of the days in Berkeley in the 1960s when they used to pass a joint around. The order and predictability of class had been replaced by total and hilarious improvisation, the practitioners having taken over the space, requesting, insisting, demanding what their all-of-a-sudden Gumby-doll bodies wanted to do.

This is what I think about teaching. It is a lot like the improvisation practiced in the playing of jazz that Winton Marsalis eloquently describes. Like jazz, teaching yoga is part solo, part swing, and part working with the blues. As with playing the trumpet, it starts and ends with the breath. This is what those who come to my classes teach me, show me, catapult me into. When I am open and relaxed and listening to what people need and are feeling inspired to do, a whole other level of yoga opens up—a joy-based playfulness done with alignment we all knew as children, that we can all find again as adults.

Creating Play Space

I recently heard a gutsy talk by David Johnson, who codirects a trauma center in New York City where he and his colleagues see many people who have not found help elsewhere—some of the most traumatized people around.[28] In this talk he spoke about a little boy, Billy, who was brought into the clinic by his foster mother, who had lost all sense of authority and connection with Billy. Johnson first met Billy wreaking havoc in the waiting room. Billy was bounding off the couches, throwing magazines, jumping on lampshades, as everyone else in the waiting room had dropped their heads into their reading material, hoping that Billy would disappear. At this point, Johnson ushered Billy and his shell-shocked foster mom into his office, where Billy threatened to upend a file drawer of forensic evidence that Johnson had recently meticulously organized. Johnson, with the biggest voice he could muster, blustered Billy and his foster mother into another room with wall-to-wall carpet, where the therapist shut the door and then stared at Billy until Billy looked up and said, "now what?!"

Johnson said, "run," at which point Billy ran lap after lap, around the perimeter of the room, with Johnson and the foster mother trailing behind, Johnson mimicking the sounds of a monster. Billy, clearly loving that Johnson was so out of "therapist" character—that he was acting a little bit like a mad man himself—kept running until he eventually plopped down on pillows, and finally got quiet enough to where the three people could start to hear each other. Although Johnson told this story for therapists who work with trauma survivors, much may be helpful for yoga teachers as well.

Trauma reduces the play space in people's lives. We need to help create play spaces for children and adults. Yoga can be a form of play. It doesn't always have to be serious. Being irreverent, breaking with protocol, running around the yoga studio, speaking with a booming rather than soothing voice may also make a space playful sometimes. Here are some other suggestions:

- Talking about "creating a safe space" often makes trauma survivors more rather than less anxious. Better to just do it, even if that requires idiosyncratic methods.

- If the trauma survivor starts to tell you something terrible she or he has lived through, move forward with your body, not back. Survivors sense body language. You might say you are up for hearing a story but if you physically back away, the survivor will back up, too.

- Trauma survivors don't want our stories told wrong, pieces left out. Accuracy matters. Remembering details matters. Being a witness to the details matters. Yoga teachers can use the skills we have honed in memorizing the dialogue for postures and sequences for remembering details of people's stories, too. We can be great listeners.

- Traumatized people are upset. People can survive being upset. Many healers are taught to hand someone a tissue as soon as they start to cry, which may signal, "Tears are bad; wipe them up." Perhaps it is better to just let them flow sometimes, snot and all.

- There is a long history of people (including health professionals) who shun trauma survivors. The Confederate General Robert E. Lee recruited many soldiers to patrol the back of fighting lines to shoot the deserters. Healers need to be careful not to shoot the survivors—by backing away from their stories; switching into problem-solving gear right away; or confusing the pain of the original trauma with the pain of retelling.

- The single factor that is most successful in keeping miners alive when they are buried beneath the earth is the belief that someone will come and rescue them, that they have not been forgotten. That is why the first thing that rescue workers do is send down a plumb line and pipe-in sound so that the miners know there are people above ground working to save them. The first thing healers need to do is let people know they will not be left alone, their story will not be forgotten.

- The number-one way for parents, teachers, therapists, and healers to not deal with trauma is to not be willing to talk about it.

The Human Spirit Is a Wondrous Thing

After a recent yoga class I taught at a community center in Boston, I found myself marveling at the human spirit. When I asked people if they had any injuries or anything they might want to celebrate about their bodies, one of the students who is in his late sixties said that his body was in good shape but he had a broken heart. He asked me if I could fix it? When I asked him how long his heart had been broken he just smiled, letting me know he was teasing. The woman next to him, whom he has known for years, kidded him that she hadn't had a chance to break his heart yet. He winked at her. Another woman said she wanted to celebrate that she could still fling her body around freely, modeling that for all of us with her arms dancing high in the air as I flashed on the glorious lyrics to an early Sweet Honey in the Rock song, "Fling my arms wide / in some place of the sun."[29] Another student, a man in his seventies who is almost completely deaf, smiled easily through the introductions and then modeled his poses on what he witnessed around him.

Most of these students won't get specific about their age. Most come to the 6 a.m. class before the yoga class—a 55-minute "Bust the Gut" class taught by the program director, who is perhaps one-third of the students' ages. After the yoga class this group will take the "Extreme Challenge" aerobics class taught by a body-building woman in her thirties who tells me that these elders set the bar so high that she simply doesn't take excuses if, in other classes, the young ones tell her they can't do it. All of the people in my class, Caribbean-born, African American, Asian American, and white, have seen their share of joy, grief, change, trauma in their lives. They tell me that what they like the most is learning the more advanced postures. The one with the playful broken heart asked at the end of class how he could improve his already sturdy balance. The dancing woman suggested that he practice tree pose (vrksasana) while waiting in bank lines or at the grocery store. I can just see him doing that.

After class, the woman who has had a yoga practice for many years tells me she is looking for a new yoga teacher to work with her daughter who is in a chair and has cerebral palsy. She tells me, "my daughter likes handsome tall men especially," if I happened to know of any yoga instructors who fit that bill. She tells me her daughter likes locust pose *(salabhasana)* the most, when she is lying on her stomach and reaches her legs and arms toward the sky. She can do cat and cow stretches, too, with support. The woman tells me that, although her daughter is thirty-two years old chronologically, developmentally she is about four. "Not a bad age to get stuck in," she tells me, "if you are going to get stuck somewhere."

The human spirit is a wondrous thing. May all people get to breathe, dance, stretch, laugh, and hold hands during tree pose (vrksasana) at some point during their lives, while sitting in wheelchairs or standing up together. May we all get to experience aging as these elders are, letting go of work as they embrace life. May there continue to be affordable, energy-filled spaces where all kinds of people can move their bodies together. May these spaces multiply.

All of Us In This World

Part of what I appreciate about yoga is its potential to make room for everybody. A recent issue of *Yoga Journal* has a two-page photo of Eric Brown, an African American aerospace engineer whose night job is to teach yoga.[30] In the photo he is in full lotus pose *(padmasana)* with Converse sneakers, a closely cropped goatee, and a finely designed buzz cut, sitting in front of a vintage airplane, its propellers doing their own symmetrical pose. On the following page is a photo of a short white woman in sailor pants and a silver vest, smiling from her warrior I pose (virabhadrasana I), perched on top of a school bus she drives during the day, teaching yoga at night. These photos remind me of one of the teachers at my home studio who, when she first started teaching, had a nose ring and a red mohawk hair cut. Five years later, her haircut is shockingly "normal" but she now has several tattoos on her arms, geometric shapes that elaborate her sculpted biceps. Audrey is a talented yoga teacher, although several of us have told her that if she ever considers a night job, it should be as a standup comedian since no amount of concentration or focus can stop people from laughing out loud once she launches into her dharma-comedian talks during practice.

Today, Audrey tells a story about one of her illustrious housemates (whom we have heard about before) who has two Chihuahuas—Sherman and Alex. We learn that Sherman is over fourteen pounds, which in Chihuahua-land is mighty big. Sherman seems okay with his size and is known around the block as a good neighbor. According to the owner, however, Alex, the smaller of the two by several pounds, is also a good dog, except for when he sees children. And except for when there is food around. And except when he is walking in the neighborhood. And except for when there are other dogs around. Except for when he is awake, with people, with other animals, or left alone. Audrey rightfully brings up to her housemate that there seems to be a lot of exceptions, a reality that brings Audrey right to the edge of self-righteousness until she sees the parallel in her own life. Telling on herself, she explains, "See, people might describe me as a patient person in general, except for when I am stressed out, except for when I am driving, except for when I am tired, or hungry, or late for work, or bored."

Her story asks us to consider how we might be able to practice patience (or self-acceptance) in ways that are the rule, rather than the exception lest we end up like Alex—a very nice dog except for, basically, all of the time. Her story also makes me think about how important it is to leave the yoga doors open for everybody, perhaps especially for bus drivers, Converse-wearing, *anjali mudra*–practicing aerospace engineers, and people sporting nose rings. Healing this world starts with recognizing all of us in the world. Even bad Chihuahuas. Walking around the block with each other. Practicing. Listening for *dharma* talks that bring laughter into the air, into our lungs, into our ways of being together.

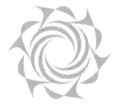

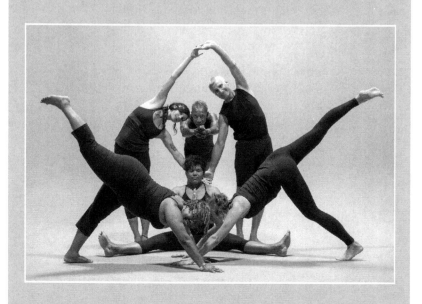

PART VI

"Love Calls Us to the Things of This World"

Yoga and Activism

What excites me most about yoga in this century is how the practice can fuel social justice—and vice versa. People around the globe are using yogic principles for all kinds of public activism—creating sustainable farms; teaching hip-hop and yoga in communities riddled by violence; using the practice to work with war-haunted refugees. Sometimes doing justice work means getting noisy, filling the streets with banners and signs, being willing to occupy for change. But sometimes, it can mean simply serving as a silent witness, keeping vigil, until the moment finally arrives when action can bring about change.

While such commitments respond directly to twenty-first-century injustices, this work has its roots in the ancient yoga traditions practiced by the *sramanas*, sixth-century BCE wonderers and wanderers who questioned established doctrines—laws, religious assumptions, social mores—while asking deep questions about what it means to be human.[1] They practiced civil disobedience of their time, and are linked to the rebels and activists in our own.

Many stories in this section reveal how yoga can bring peace to the world. Lisa Houston, a Scottish woman who has been working with Burmese refugees for many years, explains how yoga has been a lifeline for her and her family. The historian Robin Kelley describes how his mother has practiced meditation to find a peaceful state of mind even as she works against many injustices facing people in her community. Yoga is not just an interior practice. As the Buddhist writer and activist Rosa Zubizarreta tells us, "Buddha left his father's castle // to learn about //the suffering of the world."[2] This is what yoga often asks us to do, to make peace in our own castles (our bodies, homes, and communities) and also to respectfully carry our mats to where injustices exist.

In an autobiographical essay on yoga and meditation, Silvia Boorstein looks back on her decades-long work as an activist and yoga practitioner. "I am more zealous than ever about social activism. I see my activism as an aspect of spiritual practice, the natural result of being less frightened, as well as a sign of liberated energy available for purposes other than just keeping myself going."[3] There *is* something about practicing yoga and meditation over the long run that makes people less frightened. And this can be healing for trauma survivors.

Boorstein's testimony speaks to how practicing the limbs of yoga can free energy we need to do this work. And it reminds us that we must avoid what is referred to as "bypass spirituality"—the temptation to disconnect from the world and ignore its injustices on the way to personal enlightenment. Moving beyond bypass spirituality starts by recognizing that yoga communities are not immune to racism or sexism or colonialism. Creating justice within our own communities can become part of our daily practice, on our individual mats and in the work we do together.

In the end there can be no real enlightenment without an acknowledgment of the forces that divide us from one another, no inner peace without striving to create peace for everyone. I believe that yoga studios can be places that encourage us to ask deep questions about spirit and justice, as Richard Wilbur tells us in his poem "Love Calls Us to the Things of this World."[4]

Dreaming Out Loud

> Call me utopian but I inherited my mother's belief that the map to a
> new world is in the imagination, in what we see with our third eyes
> rather than in the desolation that surrounds us.
> —Robin D. G. Kelley[5]

Historian Robin D. G. Kelley opens his book *Freedom Dreams* with a
portrait of his mother: "My mother has a tendency to dream out loud. I
think it has something to do with her regular morning meditation. In the
quiet darkness of her bedroom her third eye opens onto a new world, a
beautiful light-filled place as peaceful as her state of mind." But, as Kelley
tells us, while his mother's third eye is on a place of bliss, her two other
eyes never let her forget what the people in her immediate neighborhood
are up against—"cops, drug dealers, social workers, the rusty tap water,
roaches and rodents, the urine-scented hallways . . . in a battered Harlem/
Washington Heights tenement."[6]

Kelley and his mother both know that we need the third eye to be able
to "dream out loud," because it is through the dream of freedom, through
the ability to imagine something better, that we find the strength to fight
for it. The list of wrongs to be righted—people blown up by car bombs,
children going to school hungry, little girls and boys being sexually abused
by relatives, drug addiction, the everyday violence of racism, poverty,
homophobia—is a long one. And meditation doesn't mean ignoring
social ills. Rather, Kelley believes, it shows us the way toward freedom. It
is our right, he says, our business, even our responsibility, to reach toward
freedom by dreaming it. Making our way to the land of solutions starts
with knowing that the motion toward freedom lives within us.

So what is it about practicing the postures, meditation, and mindful
breathing that can lead us to a place of freedom, not just as individuals
but also as communities? How can standing on a mat stretching your
body in multiple directions help undo the wrongs of the world? How can
sitting quietly, alone by an altar, help contribute to a less violent world?

What these processes do is unclutter our minds, help us to free ourselves from entrenched patterns of thought. Given a chance to step back, to regroup, to escape the ruts in our thinking and actions (samskaras) that have prevented us from acting in the past, we can envision new, hitherto undreamed-of solutions for the future.

If, as the Cuban American Sota Zen priest Hilda Gutiérrez Baldoquín indicates, "it is the nature of oppression to obscure the limitless essence, the vastness of who we are—that the nature of our mind is luminous, like a clear pool reflecting a cloudless sky,"[7] then yoga practice can, by changing people's thought patterns, offer us possibilities of limitless vision. Whereas oppression teaches people to think small, act small, be small, dreaming from our third eye opens a way to think big, act big, be big.

"I Fold My Blanket under Me"

> Our practice, slowly, carefully, becomes who we are. And we become
> our practice.
> —Geri Larkin[8]

In *Finding Freedom: Writings from Death Row,* the Buddhist author and San Quentin inmate Jarvis Jay Masters writes about a time when he intervened to save the life of a gay man who was about to be stabbed by another prisoner. In San Quentin, Masters explains, a gay man who is new to prison life, particularly an effeminate gay man, is at great risk of being murdered. The gay man, who looked like a woman, had walked into the exercise yard, seemingly unaware of the danger he faced. Masters, who had taken Buddhist vows to do no harm, and to stand in the way of harm being done, recounts how his mind went blank when he saw a friend of his approaching the gay man with a blade in hand: "I didn't have time to be scared, or even to think. I just knew I had to get there first."[9]

Spontaneously, he found himself acting out of depths of courage that he didn't know he had, kneeling in front of the gay man and pretending he was bumming a cigarette from him in order to put his own body between the man and his assailant. In the process he saved two lives—that of a man he did not know, and that of the man who intended to stab him, who might have been shot to death by officers in the guard tower.

Masters, a man who suffered tremendous trauma as a child and has witnessed more than a lifetime's worth in prison, offers a brave example of how meditation and mindfulness can lead to a place of justice, even when fear threatened to overwhelm him. As a man who is innocent of the crime that resulted in his death row sentence, Masters has every reason to let bitterness overtake him. Instead, he emanates hope and kindness.

It's not possible to know exactly what we would do if called upon to put our bodies in the line of fire, to intervene at the threat of a knife, a bullet, a blow. But Masters did put his body there, even while knowing that he could not possibly put an end to all the brutality of prison life. "I can't stop it," he writes. "There are stabbings every day in this place. All I have is my spiritual practice. Every morning and night I fold my blanket under me and meditate on the floor of my cell."[10]

May we all place our knees beside his, feel his courage, move from that place.

Monkey Mind

A writer's heart, a poet's heart, an artist's heart, a musician's heart, is always breaking. It is through that broken window that we see the world; more mysterious, beloved, insane and precious for the sparkling and jagged edges of the smaller enclosure we have escaped.
—Alice Walker[11]

I am attending a weekend-long workshop at Kripalu where the teacher asks us to make a list of ways that we work with monkey mind, how we move away from tricks of self-sabotage, distraction, and insecurity. Even though I am supposed to be making a list, I immediately wonder how the racing thoughts started to be called "monkey" mind. For years now, I have been unable to shake the image I saw on a documentary about scientific research on a monkey who was strapped down, day after day, as scientists performed a battery of tests on him. There was something about how his arms were splayed out, and the lack of tension in his muscles, that suggested he had finally stopped resisting. There was a look in his eyes, such a terribly defeated, sad look of resignation, puddles of disappointment. I vowed then that I wouldn't use the expression "monkey mind" to describe when my mind is running, thinking that at least my mind gets to run, isn't being drugged, isn't tied down.

The negative connotations associated with monkey mind make me think about how, in some of the literature on post–traumatic stress, there is an assumption that healing requires training our minds away from old, negative, upsetting images—that part of our work is to guide ourselves from painful associations. In this instance, such training might be to guide myself away from the image of the splayed monkey, to help my mind go to other places instead. But then I think maybe there is a reason that our minds hold onto certain images. Maybe there is something to be said for the image remaining in the front drawer of my mind—a reminder of the cruel way humans treat animals in the name of science, a reminder of how eventually it is possible to destroy a sentient being's spirit when pushed too far one too many times, that people are capable of acting as if all is okay even as they are being vicious.

In other words, while it may be helpful to replace old, damaging images with current ones of kindness and love—so that we are not run by our minds—maybe the more important lesson is to develop compassion for where our minds do go, coming to love that our minds store all kinds of images. And that some of these images have the potential to keep us humble, watchful of cruelty, cognizant that we need to be witnesses and speak up against it. I never did like the expression "monkey mind," or another, "tie the puppy to the post"—a common saying among people learning how to quiet their thoughts. I never did like leashes. I still don't.

The Mountaintop

I know that true planetary healing can only happen once we stop living the myth of separation: separation of nations, separation of races, separation of classes, separation from spirit.
—Konda Mason[12]

What does it mean to live a justice-seeking, spiritual life? Is a spiritual life different for those of us who have lived through trauma than those who have not? These questions are difficult because, of course, those who have faced a lot of hardship have more in common with those who have managed to escape major loss than not. In addition, just as all of us are only temporarily able-bodied, since all of us will eventually become less able in our bodies, the same may be true for trauma—it can be a random act that no one is immune from entirely. But there is something about trauma that enables people to ask deep questions that carry spiritual import and are linked to justice: why do bad things happen to good people, especially children? What is the nature of suffering? Are there steps to avoid suffering? How can I nurture joy? What work do I need to do in this world to make the most of the blessings I have been given, to heal myself and the earth as well?

I think about people whom I have looked to over the years for spiritual guidance, aware that one of the qualities they have in common is a willingness to talk openly about injustices. The tone of Martin Luther King Jr.'s "mountaintop" speech, the emotional waver in his cadence, let all of us know that, while he might not get there with us, he had seen the mountaintop. The power in that speech was in the intimacy of this message—he had faced down a fear of death in his willingness to stand alongside the sanitary workers in Memphis, the Vietnam vets, the old people deserving a right to vote, poor people needing steady jobs. His years of prayer (a particular form of meditation) were crucial in the wise leadership he offered.

I think too of one of my mentors Dr. Reverend Katie Cannon, the first Black woman to be ordained in the Presbyterian Church in the United

States and one of only a few African American women to teach at Episcopal Divinity School in Boston. She used to say during class she had to imagine the community of textile-working people she came from, in Kannapolis, North Carolina, in the classroom with her to be sure that she carried their concerns and joys as she spoke. Aware that so many working people, people of color, have never had access to the classrooms where she was now teaching, she carried their messages with her on her back, on her tongue, in the lessons she passed on. The injustices she had experienced—sexual abuse, racism, class elitism—is partly what led her to teach courses on liberatory social ethics. The passion, the prana in her lectures—which drew scholars and teachers from all over the country— had come through the fire of trauma, found itself on the other side, with her preaching like nobody else.

My friend Diane looks each morning to her forbearers who made it through the Middle Passage (the forced transport of Africans from their communities across the Atlantic ocean on prison ships), asking her if she is living a life that honors her journey. As an intellectual, she finds herself turning to a range of people for spiritual guidance—to Nina Simone, Mahalia Jackson, Bernice Johnson Reagon, Bonnie Raitt, Gil Scott-Heron—all spiritual people willing to sing about the wounds of the world. Our spiritual teachers don't need to be alive to still be instructing us. In fact, some of the most powerful voices are those who have passed on but have left messages for us to hear, and pass on in turn.

Long-term yoga can be one powerful way to channel the inspiration of those who have been willing to tell us about the mountaintop.

"If All Are Free to Love"

Of the yogi activists I have met and worked with over the years, one of the most compelling is Lisa Houston, a Scottish woman living on a sustainable farm in northern Thailand. Lisa is a mother of two, a devoted wife, and a poet who has been working for fifteen years with refugees on the border of Burma and Thailand. I met her when I was teaching a writing and yoga workshop, she the student, me the teacher, although those roles quickly dissolved. Her words on the page were living jewels, her generosity to the other participants in class invited an intimacy among us that inspired people's finest written work. In the morning yoga classes I taught before the writing session, her practice was a graceful weaving of breath and space, her work on the mat a centering presence. I watched as she intertwined her own body with her four-year-old daughter's on the mat, letting her daughter stretch out with her in pigeon pose (eka pada raja kapotasana), wrapping herself up next to her mom with a sarong during savasana.

In 2001 Lisa began working with a women's organization operating in nine refugee camps on the border of Thailand and Burma. Although they are officially called refugee camps, that is a misnomer since for many people, that has been their only home. Either they were born and raised there or they have no way to go back to their villages since they were burned or destroyed by the government. While doing this community work, Lisa met and fell in love with a Burmese activist, Rocky, who became her husband. Although Lisa started doing yoga on her own when she was nine—getting up into headstand and reading a book for twenty minutes at a time just because it felt good—her official foray into yoga began once she was working with a Karen (Burmese) women's organization.

Lisa started practicing yoga with a French woman, and when an Australian friend visited, she would show Lisa new postures. At that point, they designed their practice from DVDs since they didn't have a teacher. During her first pregnancy, Lisa found herself craving yoga, realizing that it was a huge shock to her system to shift from having her body to herself to needing to share. After her son's birth, she continued practicing yoga, explaining, "there is a lot that is wonderful about being a mom, but they want your body all of the time. Yoga was a way to get back into my body, to claim my body again." After she gave birth to her second child, Lisa and her friend created "For Moms and Others," a lively yoga class for people in the community and their children.

Meanwhile, as Lisa's practice deepened, she began working at a clinic serving thousands of people a year with the bare minimum in resources, treating people with all kinds of illnesses, including blackwater malaria. When this clinic was first set up in 1989, people thought that within six months the refugees would be able to go back to their communities. Fifteen years later, the clinic had become a hospital and the staff increased, as people are still not able to return to their homes.

As yoga became a mainstay for Lisa, she sought more training when she visited her family in Scotland while adding pranayama and more discipline to her routine. As she explains, "yoga is a way of clearing my mind. Before I started being able to meditate, I could put my mind on my knee, my shoulder, my hip, and ankle more easily than onto my breath. When you are an activist, your mind is racing all of the time. How do you do this? How do you learn that? You've got to be here and there at the same time, while dealing with anger all of the time at the institutions that created this situation to begin with. Yoga brings you back to yourself and your body. And you can do it anywhere."

Yoga also cushioned Lisa's husband, and so both of them, through narrow passages in their lives. By the time they moved to a farm, Rocky was suffering from deep depression and was having difficulties with drinking. He was living with the trauma of having to flee his home several times as a child and missing his father, who had been shot in the head by the military. Rocky had also been detained and harassed by the police many times. He was frozen in his own experience, angry about the terror that his people had suffered.

Eventually, Rocky and Lisa attended a yoga retreat at the International Women's Partnership for Peace and Justice, where they were able to focus entirely on yoga and healing. After they returned to the farm, Lisa would get Rocky out of bed and lead him to the yoga mat so that he would then get into the rhythm of life. After years of trying so many other things—"from not leaving his bed, to an experiment with a noose, to all kinds of traditional cures, to trying to embrace the violence of the front line, to being drunk among landmines and guns, and to making a fairly feeble (upon reflection) attempt at domestic violence—finally he was feeling okay with himself, his breath, his body and his surroundings, his weird transnational family. But it was such a complex path to get there."

Making sense of the complexity of yoga and activism, Lisa offers a story: "A friend wrote a poem for our wedding and it has sat in our room since then. One of the lines is something like—'If all are free to love, why is freedom so difficult, and he in your arms will reply it isn't, but we make it so. . . .' To me, yoga is a marvelous expression of that freedom; we are all free to do it, because it needs nothing more than us, and yet I understand why it is so difficult to get that freedom." For many activists, freedom is blocked by external forces—governmental repression, not being able to leave refugee camps—as well as internalized forces, including addiction and depression. Activism for yoga practitioners, then, is being willing to make changes on multiple levels—struggling against injustices while finding support as they get free of addictions.

The people who live on the community farm along with Lisa and her family have self-sustaining lives—growing vegetables, caring for children, building their own houses. But she knows that the people she worked with in the camps don't have those freedoms. "The stresses people have to deal with are nonstop. Sexual violence, villages being burned down, military rape." A Burmese activist woman Lisa worked with had no papers to travel in her own country. It was safer for her to live at the office where she worked since, without an ID card, traveling back to her home might risk arrest. The yoga mat was the only space she could call her own. Lisa explains, "All of the Karen women I have met who are introduced to yoga get it, immediately, as a space for them to stretch, breathe. Open up."

The Land of Infinite Possibilities

When my friend Ginger Norwood visited a few years ago while she was en route from finishing her training as a Buddhist minister in Texas back to her home in Thailand, I got the delectable chance to talk with her about her meditation and justice work.[13] During a late afternoon conversation around Jamaica Pond in Boston, I asked Ginger how she saw her mind changing during the eight-day silent retreat she had recently attended. One of her observations is that by the fifth day of silence, while she was still having thoughts, she didn't feel as bombarded by them. It was as if there was a clear pool at the bottom of her thoughts. When she did have new thoughts, they came in a more distilled way and more slowly than they had before. This allowed her to "see" the thoughts better.

While practicing silence, she had a bigger sense of possibility than before, which helped her understand her next steps. For the past decade, as the cofounder of the International Women's Partnership for Peace and Justice, Ginger has been working closely with Burmese activists, many of whom are in exile in Thailand. Hundreds of thousands of Burmese people are now living in Thailand, many working diligently for human rights in Burma. Over the years, the retreat center has been a place of regeneration, but many cannot get there since they can't use public transportation without the threat of being fined, harassed, or arrested.

Meanwhile, in recent years, Ginger has watched as the democratic struggle has taken a toll on those in exile. The resettlement policies have led to thousands of people leaving refugee camps in order to emigrate to other parts of the world—including to the United States. While this resettlement has opened some possibilities for people, those who go often feel they are abandoning both their struggles and the land that is their own in Burma. Those who stay also can feel abandoned by those who have left. Ginger has watched as many of her friends have struggled with depression, breakdown, and illness, not knowing the next steps in their work.

During the meditation retreat, Ginger saw a new possibility for her work that would include creating a center close to the border of Thailand and Burma where people could rest and recover. She would be extending the Buddhist center in Chiang Mai north, using the skills and model that she and fellow founder Ouyporn Khuankaew have been developing. Before the silent retreat, all the reasons why a satellite center might not work would flood her—making such dreams feel unrealistic if not impossible. Her exposure to secondary trauma during these last years, as a witness to the refugees' stories, had constricted her thinking. This time, optimism trumped the challenges. And she found herself less attached to the outcome—whether it would work—and more focused on its potential.

The sense of possibility that Ginger experienced firsthand has been documented recently by neuroscientists in their study of the impact of mindfulness and meditation on the brain. During trauma a sense of possibility becomes constricted as the stress hormone, cortisol, floods the hippocampus, cutting out essential communication between the left and the right brain. Healing from trauma includes rebuilding the right- and left-brain connection, a process that mindfulness and meditation supports. With this healing, constriction can be transformed into new imagination.[14] The mind's capacity to live in this location is, on a neurological level, what Ginger was describing about her experience on the retreat.

As I listened to Ginger talk, I couldn't help but think how remarkable the human mind is. The next time I find myself impatient during meditation, I will try to gently raise my finger to my lips, whispering to myself, "Shh, I am here watching for infinite possibilities."

Moses. Muhammad. Buddha. Jesus.

Is that Moses. Muhammad. Buddha. Jesus.
gathering up the morning dead?
—Sonia Sanchez[15]

A year after the 9/11 attacks, the poet Sonia Sanchez wrote a series of haiku poems in the form of two-line questions. As an unprecedented trauma in U.S. history, the 9/11 attacks were met first by an ethic of grace as people from all over the world came together to show support for the people of New York City, to mourn, in the words of poet Suheir Hammad, "sky where once was steel. / smoke where once was flesh."[16] The ethic of grace was manifest in ceremonies, both spontaneous and planned, often featuring photographs of the missing. Memorial altars were adorned with candles, flowers, and poems. People talked with neighbors for the first time about grieving and death. Children from Idaho to Japan wrote letters to children in New York whom they had never met. About the time immediately following 9/11, Moustafa Bayoumi, a scholar and New York resident, noted, "for a moment it felt that the traumatic suffering—not the exercise of reason, not the belief in any god, not the universal consumption of a fizzy drink, but the simple and tragic reality that it hurts when we feel pain—was understood as the thread that connects all of humanity."[17]

While the attacks brought forth precious manifestations of human kindness, we also soon witnessed ways that the ethic of grace was trumped by a politic of retaliation. This retaliation included vicious attacks on people of Muslim, Middle Eastern, and South Asian descent as well as a military response that then catapulted the U.S. into one and then two wars. As we witnessed this movement from grace to retaliation, many of us were grateful for the mat—that nondenominational space where all kinds of human beings, saints, gods, and goddesses could be honored as they did the work of "gathering up the morning dead."

One of the biggest gifts of yoga is its extension beyond religious lines to a space where god can be conceived of as the "om" that we chant together to welcome and close a practice; the feeling in the air when we are all breathing together; a particular deity people bring to the mat themselves; or a spirit that has no words, no images, no idolatry. In the Yoga Sutras, this is what Patanjali refers to as ishvara-pranidhana—reverence for a higher power—the fifth rule for living (niyama).[18] Such a big understanding of the spirit brings us back to an ethic of grace that birth, death, and tragedy can sometimes inspire. A grace we get to practice every day, without labels or ownership.

At the end of many yoga classes, including my own, we participate in chanting "om." To me, om is a universal sound for peace and justice. After our om I thank the class, with my hands in prayer (anjali mudra), whispering "namaste" to all. Attempting to cover a multitude of spiritual traditions, I then add, "blessed be," "power to the people," "shalom," "all Praises to Allah,"and "amen." This is fierce and loving work, this run around the bases.

An X Becomes a Heart

[Trauma survivors] know one another in ways that the most intimate of friends never will, and for that reason they can supply a
human context and a kind of emotional solvent in which the work
of recovery can begin. It is a gathering of the wounded.
  —Kai Erikson[19]

A few years ago, I attended a roundtable workshop at the Harriet
Tubman house in Boston facilitated by two activist poets, Alexis De Veaux
and Kathy Engel.[20] The workshop, the Lyrical Democracies Poetry Series,
was designed to encourage this marvelous multiracial group of young
leaders in Boston to create spoken word poetry. At the outset the facilitators asked everyone to say a bit about themselves. I am not sure why but I
talked about a story that the Black lesbian poet, activist, and breast cancer
survivor Audre Lorde writes about her book, *The Cancer Journals.*[21] After
her mastectomy, a cheery and bright-faced woman from the Reach for
Recovery Program came into the hospital room to give Lorde a pep talk
about ordering a custom-made false breast so that Lorde would look like
she did before the surgery. Lorde explained that she was looking at her
new self and that if she wore a false breast, other women who had survived breast cancer would have a hard time finding her and she finding
them. To this group of young people I found myself saying that when we
try to hide a secret, we keep ourselves from each other, maybe from the
people who we need the most, who will truly understand.

When one of the facilitators asked us to talk about writing concrete
poems—poems that take on certain shapes on the page—I found myself
raising my hand again, this time talking about a poem I wrote a long time
ago that is in the shape of an X—X as in "stop that," X as in "the action has
been banned," X, as in "this is prohibited."[22] I explained that one side of
the X, from left to right diagonally, was in the voice of a little girl who was
being raped. The other side of the X, from right to left, was in the voice
of the rapist. In the middle is where the two voices crossed, the little girl
taking in not only the force but also the consciousness of the rapist—his

worries, his guilt, his shame, his history. At the bottom of the page, far below the big X are the words,

I can't find me I am slipping
making puddles in the basement.

I looked around the room after I said these lines, realizing I had said more than I had planned, knowing I hadn't met any of the young people until an hour ago, worrying that I overwhelmed people with my intensity.

The next day one of the facilitators told me that in a poetry workshop later that day, "one of the young people had taken the idea of the X poem, with two voices crossing in the middle, and used it as a model to write one about him and his father. Only, when he wrote his, the X turned into a heart. Painful and beautiful." Learning about his X-turned-into-a-heart poem made me think about how art is a way people communicate across what might otherwise be unbridgeable divides, this connection an unexpected example of taking what we learn from yoga into the world. The generosity of various yoga teachers, therapists, poetry teachers, and friends in my life are the reasons difficult poetry has come out of my body and onto the page. Audre Lorde's visionary presence, even as she has traveled into the spirit world, keeps us celebrating her work. In this exchange, the young man's poem becomes a beautiful gift to the world. This is lucky "gathering of the wounded," where community on and off the mat grows.

Bliss Body and Tahrir Square

When I was first introduced to the five sheaths of the body—the physical, energetic, mental, wise, and bliss body—I found myself wondering if there might be a handbook somewhere, an article, an essay, a workshop that would teach about how to get from one sheath to the next. Which postures might I do, which meditations might I practice, chants I might memorize, that could lead me from the physical body to the bliss body, the faster the better? I imagined the sheaths to be like layers—the physical starts with the skin, the wise behind my heart, the energetic flying in and around me, the mental typically stuck in my brain, the bliss body nestled in my core, buried behind an organ perhaps, or tucked into a perfect pose.

Over time I have come to understand that just as ancestors don't operate on the same dimension of time that the living do, just as some weight is heavier than other weight, the sheaths of the body aren't chronological or linear either. Bliss can live on the surface of the skin (to which anyone who is falling in love can attest) just as the purely physical can live in the body of a Buddha (aka Siddhartha, for a long time, years in fact). Bliss can live in the mental body. This is the energy you can tap into when painting, writing a poem, delivering an embodied lecture, or living in the land of imagination.[23] The wise body can be available to us even when the physical or energetic bodies are waning, hence the deeply meditative, aware space my grandmother spent most of her time in during her late nineties, even as she could barely move her body on her own.

The interweaving of these five sheaths has led me to think of them as like the mycelium roots of a mushroom—an underground network of passageways that grow wider and deeper than the mushroom growing on the surface. The challenge is to find ways to fire up all of the mycelia roots at once, when all of the sheaths of the body are powered on at the same time. As yogi and philosopher Steven Cope writes, "As each seed [sheath] is opened and explored, our view of reality is profoundly altered, and we're drawn deeper, into the next seed. We cannot help ourselves. We want to know this subtle interior structure."[24]

Over the years, my biggest discovery about the bliss sheath is that it is an ineffable state that I cannot predict is coming, nor predict how to entice. But I know it when I feel it. I have felt bliss while making love—our two bodies so much our own and so much each other's at the same time while we both felt the sacred in the room with us. Another time when I felt bliss was in the middle of a boulevard in Cairo, Egypt, where more than 1,400 activists from forty-two countries traveled together in support of the people of Gaza who have been laboring for decades under Israeli control. Carrying a "Free Gaza" poster above my head written in Arabic and English, chanting up and down the boulevard feeling the support from Egyptians in their cars and on buses, I felt freer than I ever have in my life, in a complete state of bliss.

It didn't escape my attention that the clearest example of bliss I have experienced took place during a demonstration. It was a time when it felt like all of the sheaths of my body were illuminated. It was when I would say activism and samadhi were the same—a bringing together, a merging, between me and a sense of seeking justice in the world wrapped up in an incredible high. Also, it has not escaped me that immediately following the bliss was absolute panic as three military police picked my body up from behind, carried me several hundred yards and threw me into a pile of protesters surrounded by hundreds of riot police. As frightening as that moment was, it couldn't compare with the bliss that preceded it. I was doing exactly what I was meant to do—offering support for people who, for decades, had needed to be much braver than I am. The years of yoga and meditation were absolutely with me in Tahrir Square.

I know I am not alone among yoga practitioners whose feeling of bliss is linked to social justice work. Over the years, I have noticed that trauma survivors are often the ones leading the way. Standing up collectively against injustice, like doing yoga, can profoundly alter our view of reality and we cannot help ourselves. We want to know this state, this depth of connection—to ourselves and the world around us.

A Mysterious Pull

We don't know the reasons that propel us on a spiritual journey, but somehow our life compels us to go. Something in us knows that we are not just here to toil at our work. There is a mysterious pull to remember.

—Jack Kornfield[25]

In his book, *After the Ecstasy, the Laundry,* the Buddhist author Jack Kornfield asks us to find creative daily ways to see our spiritual journeys as intimately tied to other's well-being.[26] This perspective reminds me of a young woman, Nisha, whom I met in Bali when we were both completing a training in craniosacral therapy. A twenty-six year-old woman of Sri Lankan descent, Nisha was raised in Perth, Australia, by parents who held traditional expectations that Nisha would be a "proper" girl. She was constantly compared to others and asked to think and act as her parents wanted. It took her many years to understand that she could not be who her parents wanted and that she had to find her own way.

At nineteen, she studied with a talented, unconventional yoga teacher. His sometimes outlandish techniques and his huge heart—giving more than he ever could get back to the people in the studio and the whole community—gave her a yoga-inspired model for activism. At twenty-two she moved to Sri Lanka, working in a women's refuge center for young women who were pregnant or had left unsafe families. There, she taught yoga in Sinhala and English while trying to keep thirty teenage girls interested through an entire practice. Two years later, despite her parents' fury, she moved to India. There she practiced yoga with a teacher who reminded her of the Count on Sesame Street—funny, irreverent, knowledgeable. He would kill mosquitoes while announcing that it was okay since they might be enlightened in another life; he would make savasana every other pose and get everyone laughing throughout the practice.

Her early teachers helped Nisha see ways of being in the world where autonomy and quirky personalities were valued and where getting married and having children was not the only option. By the time she returned to Australia, she was no longer first her parents' child. She was her own young woman. Although she was raised in a Buddhist family based on the five precepts, Nisha did not see true compassion being practiced. Her parents had regularly used a cane to discipline her as a child, an act she thought was normal well into adulthood, when she started to say, "Hey, that was violence," and "Why would parents want to put that kind of fear into a child?" Nisha says, "When I have children, I want to hold space for them, a safe space, not physically instill fear." Now sometimes when she feels angry and finds herself lashing out like her parents did, yoga's emphasis on slowing down and meditation helps.

Through yoga she started to see a compassion she had not seen before—acceptance of many kinds of people, generosity of spirit, giving to the community without strings attached, and a bliss she would experience during and after practice sometimes that was so intense she would have to pull over to the side of the road, too high to drive safely.

Several years into her practice, Nisha still cares about the physical postures, but what matters the most is her spiritual development—her devotion to god, her wanting to practice compassion, her yearning for self-acceptance. And she wants to pass yoga onto others because it is a way to "feel alive, fully alive." She tells me, "so many people I see are dead. So much of the world suffocates people, needing to conform without thinking. In Australia, so many people live for the weekend, live for when they can drink, work jobs they don't care about. I want a different life for me and others." Like Jack Kornfield, Nisha sees a world beyond given expectations and toward serving others and ourselves.

Her continual pull toward yoga reminds me that embodied activism occurs when self-care and care for others are aligned. While some of the work transforming the world can occur with broad strokes of the activist brush—being part of a revolutionary struggle, working with Doctors without Borders, working to end violence against children—the daily commitment to be alive within ourselves is crucial as well. At twenty-six, Nisha already gets this balanced reality.

In Praise of Imperfection

... ... The only
safety lives in letting it all in—
the wild with the weak; fear,
fantasies, failures and success ...
—Danna Faulds[27]

In a remarkable dialogue that took place between Pema Chödrön and Alice Walker in San Francisco in the late 1990s, Walker said she felt incredible relief when she realized that what unites people isn't their perfection but their imperfection.[28] Perhaps, part of our work in the world is to be witnesses to each other's imperfections—for it is in that witnessing that compassion can form—tiny bubbles on the skin, a shared breath, a moment when eyes meet as tears fall. To me, compassion favors imperfection over perfection. Perfection runs the risk of being stony, off limits, stand-offish, already finished. Imperfection is much more about a process, accessible, a bridge between people to identify with each other, our foibles, limits, refusals, mistakes.

I think about a friend of mine who, while trying to quit smoking after twenty years, was keeping the imperfection of that process from me, afraid that I would judge, get angry, withdraw from her if she bumped along, bumming cigarettes once in a while, instead of going cold turkey. It turns out that her willingness, finally, to voice her imperfection helped me see better my own worries about letting addicts get anywhere close to me (since several of my relatives were alcoholics); about getting caught up in trying to "help" her; about being attached to someone who might disappear on me in a cloud of smoke; about getting distracted by her addictions and then not concentrating on my own—eating late at night, eating past full to fill a sometimes unnamable void, working too hard. It was then that compassion came into my voice, for me and for her. Compassion for my relatives who struggled with addictions and for my mother, as her willingness to keep growing and loving her three children continues.

I remember during a particularly difficult session in my first teacher training, looking up from not being able to fold forward (paschimot-tanasana), my body feeling as tight as it had when I began yoga a decade previously. While tears filled my eyes I whispered to my teacher Liz Owen, "How will I ever be a teacher if I have made no progress?" She looked at me—with wise eyes from twenty-plus years of practice—and said, "That is precisely what will make you an excellent teacher, that knowledge."

If our work in the world is about being with each other through our imperfections, that opens up a glorious, wide space for yoga, not only as a path of self-acceptance and realization, but also as a location to work for justice. Naming how the world is not perfect helps us feel our interconnectedness. The homeless man who for years has been asking for money in between traffic on a boulevard close to my house is connected to me and to my father. After my mother and father split when I was five years old, I didn't see him for many years. When we did meet again, he told me that after he lost my sister and me he "climbed on top of a mountain and drank for a long time," wandering and homeless for several periods in his life. He died at fifty-two years old, two years after he finally found sobriety, with pain pills strewn about. I see him in many people now, including in the boulevard man.

The connections among humans are often inexplicable and inextricable. The fate of a woman who recently suffocated her six-year-old son is connected to mine. She could have been me, I could have been her, when at sixteen, working as an unpaid nanny, I would shake the infant I was watching too hard, too long, sleep weary, desperate myself. I am connected to the yoga teacher I looked at rudely when she corrected me for the fourth time in one class. She and I share a predilection toward precision, even as my body caves in for the last fifteen minutes of class.

So many sages have long told us that peacefulness in oneself is a path to peace in the world. My daughter calls me from the next room wanting to go out into the sun together. I vow to leave this writing in an imperfect place, momentarily pass up my rush to finish, another symptom of an elusive striving for perfection.

This morning, I remind myself, keep contemplating about this, gently.

Making Room for Despair

I am just back from a beautiful yoga practice where only three people came, which meant we had a semiprivate session for an hour and a half, my body soaking in the teacher's subtle cues, sophisticated suggestions. I come home high and grateful only to hear that the state of Georgia had executed Troy Davis the night before, a man who, until the end, had insisted on his innocence, his initial trial a travesty of justice. Tears ache out of me, wondering how we can make sense of this act that people from all over the world had protested—the pope, Desmond Tutu, and Jimmy Carter among them. How to make sense of state-sponsored premeditated murder that thousands of people had stood up against, that was, by any measure, wrong. I call friends—people who have been working to stop the epidemic of incarceration in this country, those who have opposed the death penalty and other acts of cruelty—finding myself remembering that the noted activist Howard Zinn had once said that he made room for despair on alternate Tuesdays from 2 to 2:30. This day is my Tuesday.

And I ask: what can yoga really do to stop the cruelties we witness around us—poverty, sexual abuse, child neglect, war, the death penalty? A close friend and fellow poet and activist Randall Horton hears the sadness in my voice as we ask each other, what can poetry do? What can yoga do? What can prayer do? What can organizing do? What can anything really do? Nothing will bring Troy Davis back. Nothing seems to be slowing the abuse of children. Nothing seems to be stopping global warming. How can I, in good conscience, write a book about how yoga can help us heal from trauma, when, on this particular day, I cannot say how yoga helps?

The great Chilean poet Pablo Neruda once said that what scares a dictator most is the poet, a claim that makes sense given all of the poets who, through time, have been imprisoned, the passion of their words enough to justify their exile. Might yogis across time and circumstance be able to incite such prana, nurture such inner peace, practice such grounding postures that we might, even for a moment, be able to will the very first yama—nonviolence—of the very first limb of yoga, into worldwide practice? Might the idea of it be enough to start a wavelength where the taking of human life would simply be considered inconceivable? What will it take for us to make that very first yama our life's work, our life's bread? Today I ask this, in the memory of Troy Davis and all the brave, humble people who tried to make sure that he was still living and breathing with us, right now.

The Way Home Tour

There is no one path
but many
no one answer
but many
the eye of the needle
opens to an infinite
universe

I am awakened, disturbed, in the night, especially about this last section on yoga as a guide for activism, knowing that yoga communities have so much to learn. It is easy to romanticize yoga. It is so easy to fall into bypass spirituality. So easy to offer yoga retreats all over the world that reproduce the same tourist relationships—wealthy Westerners going to be served by people who may not have access to yoga themselves, who may not have access to the gorgeous land many retreats have been built on except to keep it pretty for the tourists. I am up in the night thinking, too, how easy it is to turn the eight limbs into their own dogma, to start to consider these limbs *the way,* to ground ourselves only as deep as the concrete floor where the yoga studios have been built, not deeper, not into the land and people who have protected and loved the land before the yoga studios existed. This all worries me. It reminds me how yoga activism must begin from a place of humility, knowing that mindfulness, disciplined uses of the body, and meditation were practiced by people on this land way before us.

In the western hemisphere, a prayer rug I travel to psychically belongs to Don Coyhis, who is from the Mohican nation and is the cofounder of White Bison, an organization that focuses on Native American healing. Coyhis created the Wellbriety project to support Native Americans who seek to live free of addiction. He also envisioned the Forgiveness Project Way Home Tour. This 2010 project involved a group of people who traveled from Washington State to Washington, D.C., stopping at the places where boarding schools still stand or used to be, in order to do rituals of forgiveness. These "schools" which operated from 1879 until well into the 1970s, cost whole generations of Native American people their present and future—children, the continuity that makes it possible for a culture to survive.

On the tour, they were asking the forgiveness of the children whose spirits were left at these schools. There are mass graves at some of the schools, children buried with no names, given no grave stones, no visible connection to their families. On the journey, the group also granted forgiveness to the U.S. government for the atrocities committed. Even though the government has never acknowledged the devastation caused by these schools, Native American people know that they cannot wait for an apology to be offered until forgiveness is granted. The rage, confusion, and betrayal that people carry need to be released regardless of governmental negligence and abuse. Forgiveness can be offered, even when responsibility has not yet been taken.

This is a difficult message—that forgiveness is an option, even a necessity, although no apology has been made. But this is what yoga and meditation teaches. This is what can come from smudging, from listening to the mountains, from staying still. The space of stillness where the mind stops running is a space that seeks forgiveness.

There is resonance between the eight-limbed path of yoga and the Native American Code of Ethics that Don Coyhis offers in *The Red Road to Wellbriety*. For example, the first principle of the Native Code: "Rise with the sun to pray. Pray alone. Pray often. The Great Spirit will listen, if only you speak."[29] That sounds like early morning yoga, spreading your mat, beginning in child's pose (balasana), opening your practice with "om," the universal sound of union, harmony, sealing your practice with "om" again, in anjali mudra.

Another beautiful pairing: The Native American principle, "Bad thought causes illness of the mind, body, and spirit. Practice optimism." resonates with contentment (santosa, the second niyama), practicing the moment-to-moment awareness that you are okay, you are still here, are still breathing, its own daily miracle. What about the Native American principle, "Children are the seed of our future. Plant love in their hearts and water them with wisdom and life's lessons."[30] Can you ask forgiveness to the child you left behind, unsure how to care for a child who had been injured? How did that abandonment start for you? Was it when you were separated from yourself during abuse, after an accident when you were paralyzed, when you "forgot" what happened to you, lashing out from the missing memory? Was it when you tore limbs from a spider and laughed out loud when inside you wept? Was it when your anger turned to hunger, leaving you desperate for food, even when you are full? Abandonment happens during trauma—too many pieces to hold onto, too hard to find, too hard to see. The prayer rugs of the world are telling us that forgiveness is a process—meditation, prayer, listening, asanas can be daily practices to help us.

Willow on the Seine

In a recent talk, Eve Ensler, the creator of the gutsy *Vagina Monologues*, shared a part of her own story that was so poignant, so honest that I couldn't help but quote it at length:

> For a long time, there was me and my body. Me was stories, cravings, desire. Me was trying to not become an outcome of my violent past— this led me to the *Vagina Monologues*. One night on stage, I entered my vagina. Then I became a driven vagina. . . . The more I talked, the more objectified I made my body.
>
> Then I went to the Democratic Republic of the Congo. I heard stories that made me get inside of my body. Many women had holes in their bodies. . . . Then I got cancer. It arrived like a speeding bird smashing into a windowpane. Then I had a body. Cancer exploded the wall of my disconnection. . . . Before cancer I was separated from the world. Now I am swimming in it. Now I make a daily pilgrimage to visit a willow on the Seine. . . . The recipe for survival has to do with paying attention . . . 1000 prayers, a million oms.[31]

Eve Ensler's poetic and brazen love for life makes a profound link between taking care of our bodies and caring for the earth, with healing the holes in each of our souls. Her words remind me that taking risks is contagious, brilliance is contagious. Honoring the spiritual leaders, writers, activists, healers among us is part of transforming the world. Charles Johnston writes, "All true art is a contagion of feeling; so that through the true reading of true books we do indeed read ourselves into the spirit of the Masters."[32] Higher consciousness can be passed on through space, touch, asanas, in stillness. Surrounding ourselves with people whose prana is flowing, whose asana practice is dynamic and alive, whose spiritual practice allows them to exude an attitude of authenticity and grace—can keep us going, finding them in us, and us in them. Here's to a thousand prayers, a million oms.

To Carry the Sky on Your Head

> She told me about a group of people in Guinea who carry the sky
> on their heads. They are the people of Creation. Strong, tall, and
> mighty people who can bear anything. Their Maker, she said, gives
> them the sky to carry because they are strong. These people do not
> know who they are, but if you see a lot of trouble in your life, it is
> because you were chosen to carry part of the sky on your head.
>   —Edwidge Danticat[33]

In her stunning novel, *Breath, Eyes, Memory,* Edwidge Danticat writes about three generations of Haitian women who walk, fly, sing, plead, write, and love their way toward freedom. Sophie, the daughter portrayed in the novel, was birthed by a mother who had been raped by the Tonton Macoutes, a paramilitary goon squad trained by the CIA who used their muscle and systematic violence against women as a way to keep the Haitian people terrified for generations. The aunt who raised Sophie in Haiti until her stateside mother could send for her told Sophie that she was born from "the petals of roses, water from the stream and a chunk of the sky"[34]—a genesis that deliberately leaves the perpetrator out, while drawing on the healing powers of earth and sky.

Breath, Eyes Memory tells us a lot about the healing process—that we need myth, legend, and stories to help us reckon with evil. It also lets us know about many of the other resources that can help save people's lives. While Sophie's mother, who was never able to get the picture of the faceless men who raped her out of her mind, eventually kills herself, her daughter makes it to a hard-won freedom, and in fact comes to thrive by the end of the novel. Unlike her mother, Sophie had access to therapy, spiritual sustenance, loving touch, and other resources not available to her mother's generation.

Breath, Eyes, Memory teaches us about the power of collective action. When people come together, whether in social movements or healing circles, to stand up against injustice, they create sanctuaries of accountability and peace. This is what yoga communities can do, too. For millions of people, yoga is a way of stretching our bodies, tuning into our own breath and heartbeats, and finding a much-needed physical release. But it can be something more, too. Within the sound of our breath and our heartbeats we may sometimes find ourselves listening to our soul's prayers. And that can take us to a different place, where embodied practices lead to embodied principles, and from there to a social activism that could even, ultimately, involve putting our own bodies on the line.

I close this book with Danticat's quote because it teaches us why doing headstands and handstands is a good idea. During the time you are inverted, you get a rest from carrying the sky on your head. Until, of course, you put your feet on the ground again, renewed and refreshed, with newly found prana to carry you forward.

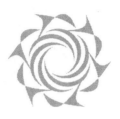

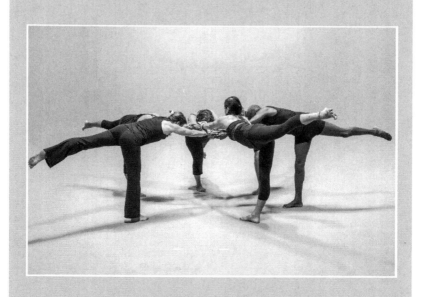

APPENDIX I:
THE EIGHT LIMBS OF YOGA

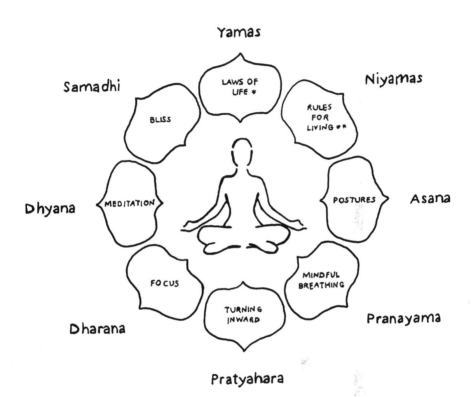

Yamas

Samadhi

LAWS OF LIFE *

Niyamas

BLISS

RULES FOR LIVING **

Dhyana

MEDITATION

POSTURES

Asana

FOCUS

MINDFUL BREATHING

TURNING INWARD

Pranayama

Dharana

Pratyahara

* Laws of Life
Nonviolence (ahimsa)
Truthfulness (satya)
Integrity (asteya)
Sexual Accountability(brahmacharya)
Nonattachment (aparigraha)

** Rules for Living
Simplicity (sauca)
Contentment (santosa)
Purification (tapas)
Self-study (svadhyaya)
Devotion (isvara-pranidhana)

Picture by Caitlin Sweeney

217

APPENDIX II:
GLOSSARY OF POSES

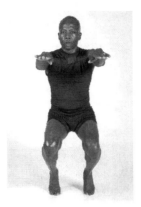

awkward pose *(utkatasana)*

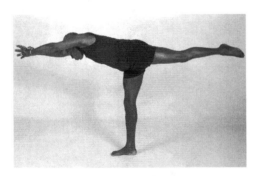

balancing stick
(tuladandasana)

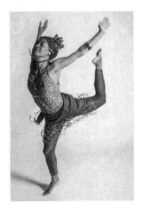

bird in flight

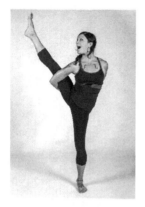

bird of paradise *(svarga dvidasana)*

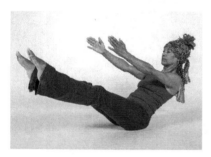

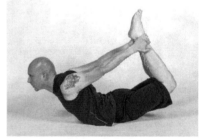

boat *(navasana)*

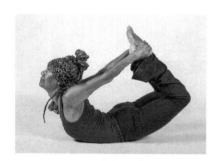

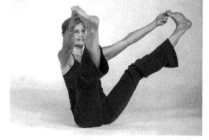

bow *(dhanurasana)*

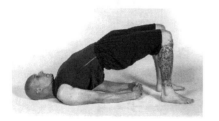

bridge *(setu bandha sarvangasana)*

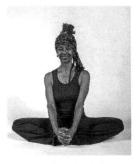

butterfly pose *(baddha konasana)*

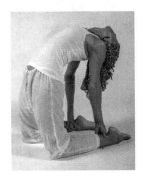

camel *(ustrasana)*

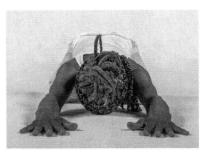

child's pose *(balasana)*

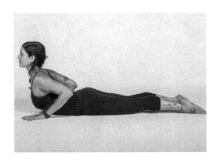
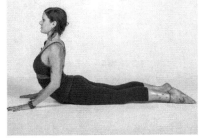

cobra *(bhujangasana)*

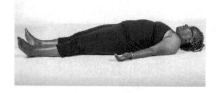

corpse pose *(savasana)*

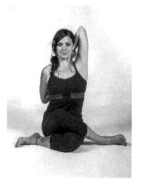
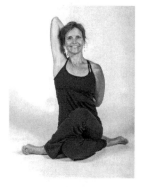

cow-face pose
(gomukhasana)

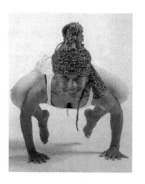

crow *(bakasana)*

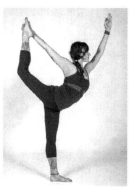
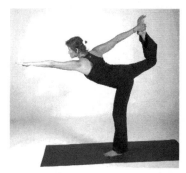

dancer *(dandayamana
dhanurasana)*

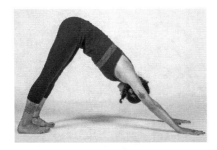

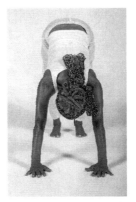

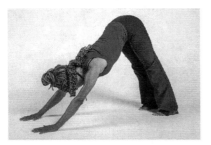

downward-facing dog *(adho mukha svanasana)*

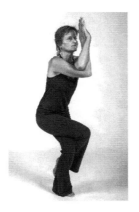

eagle *(garudasana)*

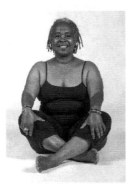

easy pose *(sukhasana)*

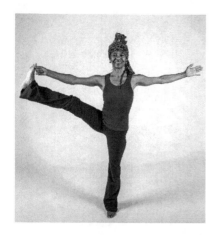

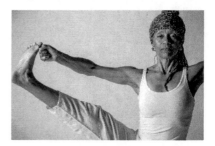

extended hand-to-foot pose II *(utthita hasta padangusthasana II)*

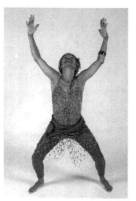

free goddess *(utkata konasana)*

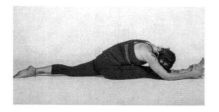

full splits *(hanumanasana)*

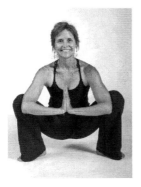

garland *(malasana)*

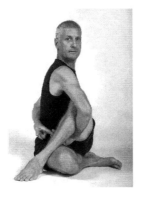

half lord of the fishes *(ardha matsyendrasana)*

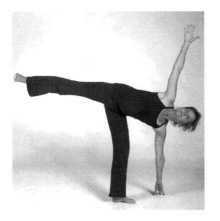

half moon *(ardha chandrasana)*

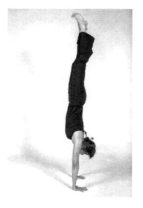

handstand *(adho mukha vrksasana)*

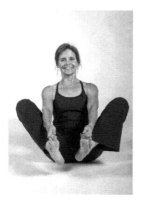

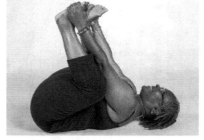

happy baby *(ananda balasana)*

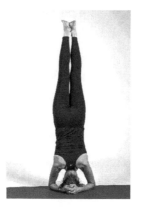

headstand *(sirsasana)*

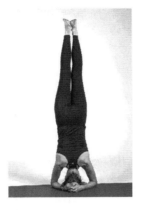
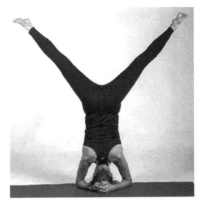

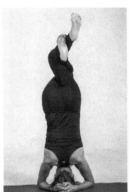
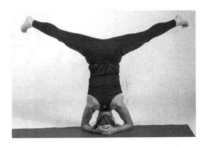

headstand cycle *(sirsasana)*

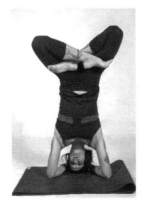

headstand in lotus
(sirsasana and *padmasana)*

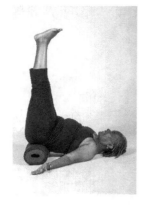

legs up the wall pose
(viparita karani)

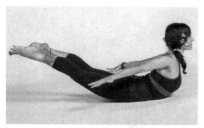

locust *(salabhasana)*

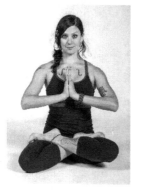

lotus *(padmasana)*

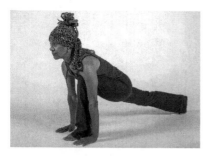

lunge

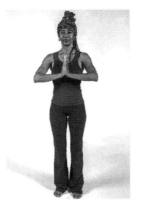

mountain *(tadasana* with *anjali mudra)*

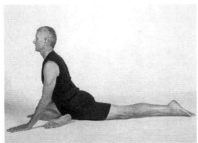

pigeon *(eka pada raja kapotasana)*

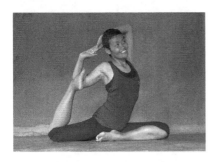

pigeon II *(eka pada raja kapotasana II)*

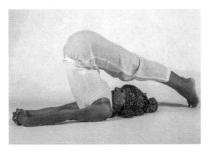

plow *(halasana)*

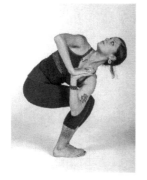

prayer twist *(parivrtta utkatasana)*

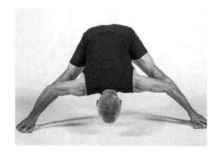

pyramid *(prasarita padottanasana)*

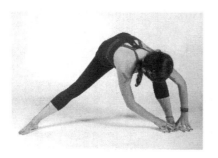

pyramid sway *(prasarita padottanasana)*

rabbit *(sasangasana)*

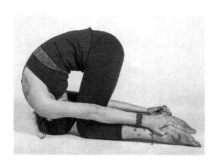

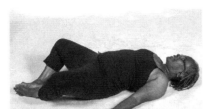

reclined butterfly *(supta baddha konasana)*

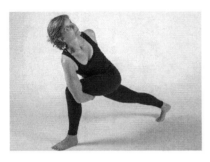

revolved bound side angle *(parivrtta baddha parsvakonasana)*

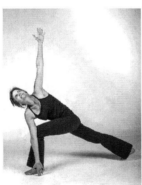

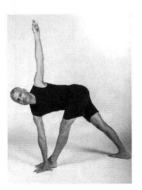

revolved extended side angle *(parivrtta parsvakonasana)*

revolved triangle *(parivrtta trikonasana)*

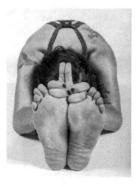
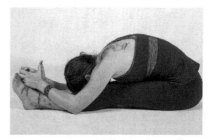

seated forward bend
(*paschimottanasana*)

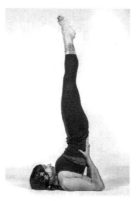

shoulder stand
(*sarvangasana*)

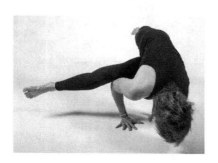
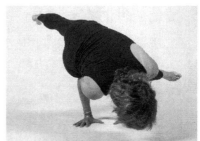

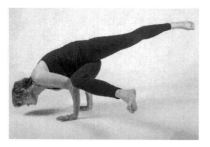

side crow (*parava bakasana*)

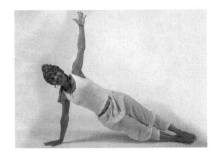

side plank *(vasisthasana)*

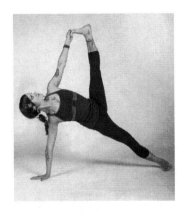

side plank II
(vasisthasana II)

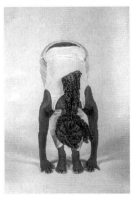

standing forward bend
(uttanasana)

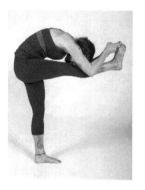

standing head to
knee *(dandayamana
janushirasana)*

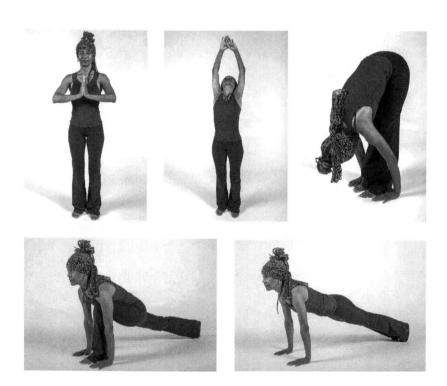

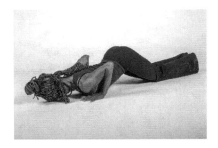

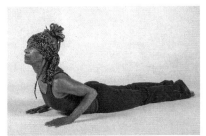

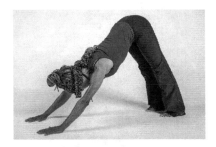

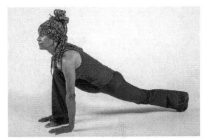

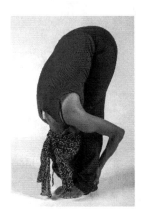

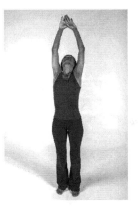

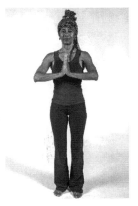

sun salutation *(surya namaskar)*

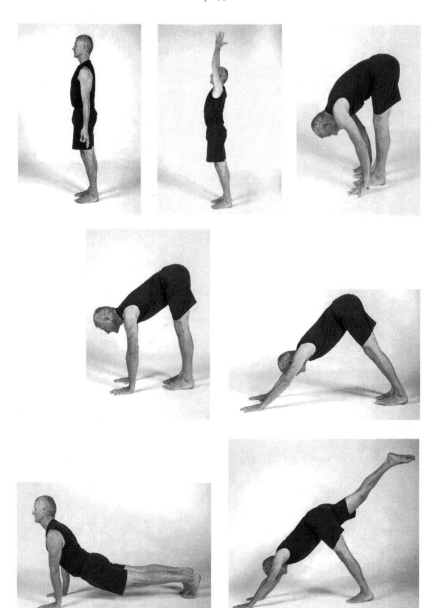

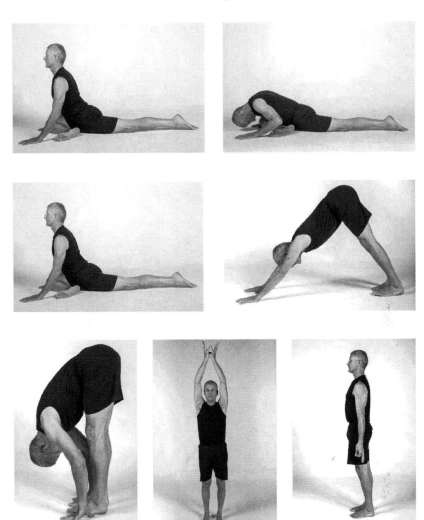

sun salutation Kali Ray style

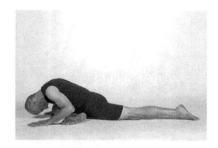

swan bow

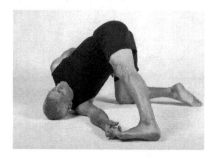

thread the needle

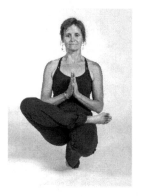

toe stand *(padangustasana)*

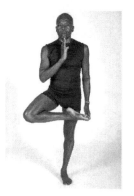

tree *(vrksasana)*

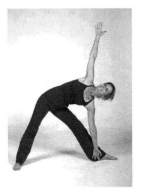

triangle *(trikonasana)*

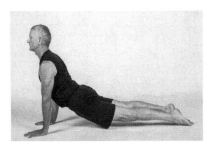

upward-facing dog *(urdhva mukha svanasana)*

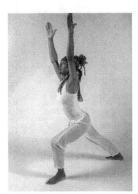

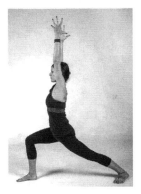

warrior I
(virabhadrasana I)

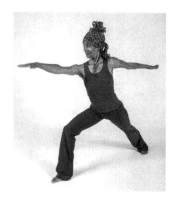 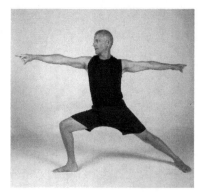

warrior II
(virabhadrasana II)

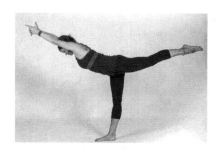

warrior III
(virabhadrasana III)

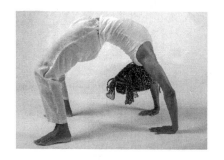

wheel *(urdhva dhanurasana)*

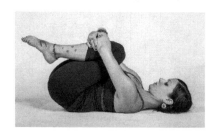

wind removing
(pavanamuktasana)

Collective Poses

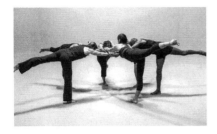

balancing stick in a circle
(tuladandasana)

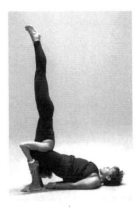

bridge meets headstand
(setu bandha sarvangasana
and *sirsasana)*

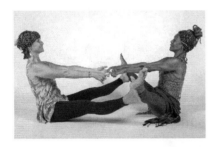

double boat *(navasana)*

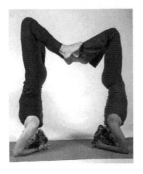

double headstands
(sirsasana)

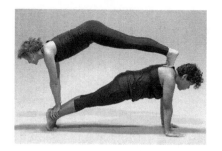

double planks

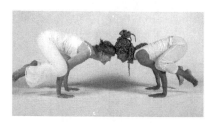

facing crows *(bakasana)*

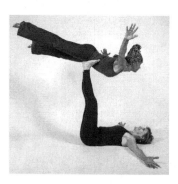

flying pose

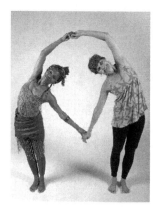

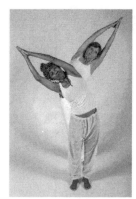

funky half moons

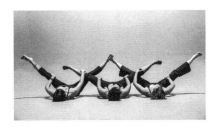

lattice *(viparita karani)*

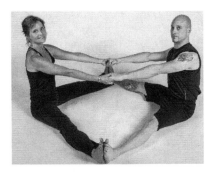

partner straddle

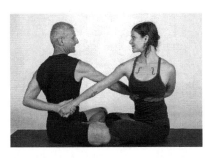

partner twists

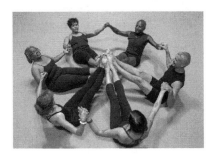

petal pose

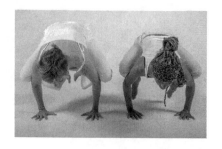

side by side crows
(bakasana)

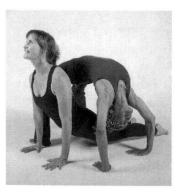

tree to forest *(vrksasana)*

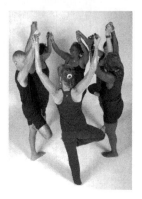

wheel and up dog *(urdhva dhanurasana* and *urdhva mukha svanasana)*

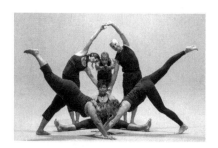

yoga party

APPENDIX III:
FINDING THE YOGA
THAT WORKS FOR YOU

While yoga's healing components are increasingly well known, making sense of which tradition of yoga is best for you can be confusing. While there is no one type of yoga that is better for trauma survivors than others, it is good to know what you are walking into. Finding the right yoga tradition and teacher is like buying new shoes. You often need to try on many pairs, even go to different stores before you find just the right fit. For example, the intensity of Bikram, Ashtanga, and Power Yoga can quickly help people shift their moods away from worry and self-doubt as the rigor of the class takes you into sensation and embodied learning. (You don't have time to be yelling at yourself since all your attention needs to go to sticking a posture.) Trauma survivors who may be flooded by emotion or flashbacks often thrive in intense classes that leave you no option but to drop your thoughts and go into your body. (The idea here is: meet the mind where the mind is so that the body and mind can release.)

For others, though, such intensity can feel scary, demanding, even suffocating. For them, the restorative elements of Yin Yoga, Slow Flows, and Kundalini can bring a welcome meditative calm. Some of the practices focus more on spirituality than others. However, even the more physical practices often lead people toward spirituality (since a deepening connection with our bodies draws us toward spirit). The range of effects of various yoga approaches is why many trauma survivors are hybrid practitioners—we seek out a range of traditions.

Personally, I am biased in favor of teachers who have been teaching for a long time, who are self-reflective (they do their own emotional, spiritual, and physical work), are humble, and are flexible (are willing to regroup and learn from students).[1] I adore classes that include music (it helps me slip away from scolding or repetitive thoughts), but there is something to be said for the music of your own breath, too. Whatever style you choose, know that you are your first and last teacher and that you deserve thoughtful, caring communication from teachers. This appendix provides brief descriptions of major schools of yoga and how they may (or may not) be helpful to you. [2]

Anusara: a complex and elegant system that combines biomechanical precision with a life affirming tantric yoga philosophy. Anusara gives attention to spirituality (in particular opening oneself to "grace") and may be especially useful for people wanting to work with the muscular and energetic body. The attention to specific cues helps survivors integrate aspiration with physical alignment (opening up to grace in that moment, in your own particular way). It may include some partner work, which can be helpful in terms of developing trust and risky if boundaries feel threatened.

Ashtanga: the Sanskrit word for an eight-limbed practice based on six fast-paced, flowing, and vigorous asana sequences that you learn sequentially (and that are increasingly challenging and cumulative). The athletic sequences are intended to build stamina and strength. The Krishnamacharya-inspired yoga, which was originally practiced and codified in Mysore, India, by K. Pattabhi Jois, is often a self-practice called Mysore-style (with some supervision) that can be useful for people who want to pace themselves and who thrive on individualized instruction. Teacher-led Ashtanga practices are highly structured and are intended to teach you the poses as perfectly as possible. The expectations can help build confidence as you progress, which can be empowering. The intensity of the practice can be tricky for survivors who already tend to push hard, but the practice of the established sequences can also provide a sense of stability and safety.

Bikram: practiced in a hot and humid room to encourage flexibility and focus. It was created by Indian-born Bikram Choudhury based on twenty-six postures and two breathing exercises performed in exactly the same order in each class. This series builds stamina and is often initially sought out by those who want a physical practice and for those with chronic injuries. (It is particularly successful for people with back problems.) It can be a powerful method for detoxifying since there is lots of sweating. The sequence tends to work well for people who appreciate predictability. The script cadence that is recited by the instructors can also quiet internal chatter. Possible limits of this practice include that there is very little room for individuality (which many trauma survivors thrive on to feel "seen"), little hands-on instruction, and almost no mention in the script to the spiritual dimensions of yoga.

Forrest: a muscular, alignment-based practice developed by Ana T. Forrest.[3] This practice is useful for trauma survivors partly because the cues are designed to keep people focused on feeling in the present time and working through energy blocks. Forrest Yoga offers much attention to core strength and the use of the breath and visualization to heal. Many Forrest-trained teachers are exquisitely attuned in their ability to offer adjustments that can facilitate welcome physical and emotional release. Perhaps because of Forrest's personal history of healing (from addiction, sexual abuse, epilepsy, and eating problems), Forrest classes make deliberate room for healing from trauma. It is a fierce practice that may be intense for people at various times in the healing process. There is also very little movement, which can feel emotionally stagnating for some people.

Iyengar: named after B. K. S. Iyengar, arguably the most influential modern day yoga master. As one of the older hatha systems, the Iyengar tradition embodies a healing power due its longevity and reliability. It uses props—blocks, straps, and bolsters—to hold poses for significant periods to help people find comfort and stability. There is an emphasis on precise alignment of challenging poses with beginner, intermediate, and advanced classes. For many people there is safety in its structure— you are taught exactly what to do and what is required, since teachers spend considerable energy working with each person's individual body.

The teachers are trained to look at practitioners energetically, looking closely at their bodies, their faces, even their skin to see what is going on inside and to stay with people in distress until their energy has calmed down. Iyengar classes are also great places to learn inversions since there is sophisticated attention to alignment and long holds. (Inversions can do wonders for mood and confidence.) The down sides of an Iyengar practice are that it can feel rigid and there is no use of flow, dance, or music.

Kripalu: an on- and off-the-mat yoga practice. The on-the-mat asana practice teaches how to remain fully present, "ride the wave" of emotions, and observe oneself compassionately. Kripalu Yoga then encourages students to apply those skills in the rest of their lives. The tradition emphasizes breath work (pranayama), which helps with emotional, physical, and mental balance. This focus can be beneficial for "living into" and healing from trauma. Because Kripalu is meant to meet everyone where they are physically, it's a good practice for those who should not force themselves into textbook asana. The spiritual interconnectedness helps people who are withdrawn or feel cut off from the world. The emphasis on compassion and individual journeys allow people emotional, physical and spiritual flexibility and permission to find their own way.[4]

Kundalini: a safe and elegant practice brought to the West by Yogi Bhajan after being handed down orally (and in secret) for thousands of years. A methodical combination of kriyas (a set of exercises), mantras, breathing, singing, meditation, and relaxation created to awaken people's creative potential. There is emphasis on spiritual development, wholeness, and devotion. It is an excellent practice for trauma survivors due to the awareness of an infinite self (the soul) that cannot be injured, that always remains. The study of Kundalini invites people to see how the finite self is in reaction to one's karma but that it is possible to act and live from a place of the soul. The repetition of chanting, mantras, and breath can transport you into expansive realms. (The use of fairly straightforward poses may also provide alternatives for those who find limits in more elaborate asanas). The "Breath of Fire," a commonly used pranayama exercise in Kundalini, helps balance the sympathetic and parasympathetic nervous system, which trauma often disturbs. One possible caution about this practice is that it can be so powerful in accessing the subtle life force that you might get overwhelmed and disoriented initially, until you learn to work with the energy in a measured way. The methodical use of mantras and breathing exercises might also feel too repetitive and staid for people who find integration in flowing practices.

LifeForce Yoga: an evidence-based approach to healing developed by Amy Weintraub for anxiety and depression and used in mental healthcare settings and therapeutic yoga settings across the globe. The approach synthesizes practices from several yoga lineages with attention to current research. The foundation of the practice is to meet the practitioners where they are and to move slowly, using breath, mudra (hand gestures), mantra, and gentle body-sensing yoga movement to allow them to reoccupy their bodies. The approach provides people with self-empowering tools to manage moods. The practice rests on the premise that within each of us is a wellspring of wholeness, where despite the traumas and losses we have lived through, we are whole. The practices provide a portal into that wholeness. The practices clear the mind's spiral of negative self-talk, providing a window through whatever mood state is visiting, to that inner sense of wholeness unsullied by the trauma story.

Power Yoga: First named by Beryl Bender Birch and Bryan Kest in the late 1980s, this hot *vinyasa* practice is not as sequentially exacting as Ashtanga, but still has an emphasis on one breath, one movement with flowing sequences. It is designed to be vigorous in order to build strength and flexibility. Power Yoga can be a great confidence builder in terms of stamina. However, its fast pace does not allow for the subtle attention to alignment that Iyengar provides. Its popularity also means there may be little individual attention during class. And, typically, there is little explicit attention to spiritual development.

Restorative: a relaxation-based practice where simple poses are held for extended periods (5–10 minutes), often with the help of bolsters and straps for maximum comfort. This yoga can be a powerful healing practice that nurtures people's relationship to stillness and silence. For some practitioners, the slow pace is a welcome way to relax. The meditative, gentle characteristics of this practice stimulate the parasympathetic nervous system, which can be marvelous for people with chronic fatigue and others who want to find deep and regenerative breath. For some, the slowness makes it hard to quiet a racing mind. A caution for Restorative Yoga for trauma survivors is that it can cause dissociation, numbness or "spacing out." Modifying poses, staying connected to the earth, and keeping your eyes open can help along with knowing that you, not the teacher, are the "ultimate authority."

Trauma-Sensitive Yoga (TSY): This approach focuses on using asana as a way to notice what we feel in our body, to practice making choices about what to do with the asana based on what we feel, and to experiment with taking action within the asana. The approach is client-centered; that is, the emphasis is on the subjective experience of each participant and not on an external value of "getting a form right." TSY was created in a clinical context at the Trauma Center at the Justice Resource Institute as a treatment for complex trauma. One limit of this approach is that, currently, it is only available in Boston. In addition, the program requires that the practitioner also be in therapy while doing the yoga program (since, when you start to pay attention to your body, you will invariably connect with implicit memories that can be overwhelming without compassionate and qualified support). The therapy requirement is especially hard for veterans who often have to wait months to get authorization for therapy and for sex workers and others who may not have any connection to therapeutic services.

Vinyasa: This popular practice, which means breathing and moving in sync, includes slow and rapid flows, often incorporating sun and moon salutations with attention to core strength. Often practiced in a hot room, the sequences are created to build stamina and experience a dynamic combination of strength and ease in postures. As a moving rather than static meditation, this approach can be particularly healing for people who have been restrained (literally or figuratively) since it is dance-like. The ability to flow provides a sense of safety, integration, and grace as the energy moves from the heart to the breath to the body. A limitation of Vinyasa is that a fast pace can leave new practitioners feeling somewhat lost since there is little individualized instruction. Vinyasa pays little explicit attention to the deeper, spiritual aspects of yoga. On the other hand, the flowing movement can feel divine if the pace, sequence, and music selection are in sync.

Yin Yoga: This approach focuses on poses that help relax the muscles and stimulate connective tissue for a variety of physical and energetic benefits. Yin yoga can bring up strong sensations and emotional patterns because you hold poses for three to six minutes. You may use props if they support your ability to deepen or stay in the pose longer. A central tenet of yin yoga is to play the edge—feeling mild to moderate stimulation but not enough to be overwhelming. A practitioner can move in or back off from a pose in service of playing that edge. Energetically, holding these poses stimulates the meridian system, which can promote emotional equilibrium. Yin can be a bitter practice with a sweet result as you are sometimes opening to and staying with challenging physical and mental patterns and then cultivating a relaxed and receptive disposition to a broad range of experience. Since yin yoga offers a meditative opportunity, it can encourage capacities of mindfulness and compassion that allow people to acknowledge and perhaps dis-identify with emotions and memories that may arise (uncoupling from the content and seeing what is coming up as a flowing process). This approach to emotional work is different than ironing out or tacking down a story—rather it is about seeing the story as a process. While the simplicity, stillness, and quiet of the practice can be deeply nourishing, for trauma survivors the emotional journey may also be threatening and overwhelming. It becomes important to work with teachers who make space for emotional reactions and who emphasize treating oneself with great kindness.

Y12SR: an innovative, life-changing, grassroots program that combines twelve-step recovery for people with addictions with yoga, founded by somatic practitioner, yoga therapist, and trauma survivor Nikki Myers. The program recognizes the cognitive value of twelve-step recovery principles with the somatic value of yoga, coupling the two for people seeking long-term recovery. The yoga instruction focuses on asana and meditation that fosters somatic awareness, balancing of the central nervous system, and emotional stability. The synergism between the cognitive and somatic approach to healing enables a powerful method of dealing with unresolved trauma, the recognition of signs of relapse, and the building of inclusive communities of accountability. This community-based platform began in Indiana in 2004 and has spread to multiple locations across the United States.

For further exploration: There are several other yoga approaches you might see advertised at studios and community centers, including: Phoenix Rising Yoga Therapy (individualized attention to physical and psychological healing); Jivamukti (highly meditative; the Sanskrit translates to "liberation while living"); AcroYoga (partner inversions and flying); Kali Ray TriYoga (flowing, dance-like); White Lotus (personalized practice); Svaroopa (means "transcendent inner experience"); Sivananda (twelve postures, chanting); and others.[5]

SELECTED ADDITIONAL RESOURCES

Below is a list of resources that have been company in the wee hours; books I keep tucked into my suitcase and draw from in workshops; music I dance to and incorporate into playlists for yoga classes.

Trauma and Healing

Ana T. Forrest, *Fierce Medicine: Breakthrough Practices to Heal the Body and Ignite the Spirit* (New York: HarperOne, 2011). A hybrid memoir and practice guide written by one of the bravest yogis, this book draws on Forrest's own intense story of healing as well as Native American, European, and Eastern wisdom to help catapult our healing forward.

bell hooks, *Sisters of the Yam: Black Women and Self-Recovery* (Boston: South End Press, 1993). Hooks is one of the most prolific women writers of her generation. This book is among her best, telling painful and honest truths about Black women's ability to heal from addictions, loss, breakups, racism. While specifically written about Black women, hook's words teach us all about healing and justice.

Amy Weintraub, *Yoga for Depression: A Compassionate Guide to Relieve Suffering through Yoga* (New York: Random House, 2004). Written by a master yoga teacher whose practice helped relieve her own depression, this book offers an accessible, hopeful, and conscientiously researched guide for people with depression and those who love them. Weintraub is also the creator of LifeForce Yoga. For more about this approach to healing and locations in your area go to www.yogafordepression.com.

Akasha Gloria Hull, *Soul Talk: The New Spirituality of African American Women* (Rochester, VT: Inner Traditions, 2001). Based on conversations with Alice Walker, Lucille Clifton, Sonia Sanchez, Toni Cade Bambara, and other luminaries, this book celebrates a renaissance of spiritual consciousness among women, a creativity that can help heal each other and the planet.

Louise DeSalvo, *Writing as a Way of Healing: How Telling Our Stories Transforms Our Lives* (New York: HarperOne, 1999). Written by a long-time creative writing professor and scholar on Virginia Woolf, this book teaches us ways that writing can be a witness and a source of regeneration.

David Emerson and Elizabeth Hopper, *Overcoming Trauma through Yoga: Reclaiming Your Body* (Berkeley, CA: North Atlantic Books, 2011). Written by two scholar healers who are directors of yoga services and Project REACH, respectively, at the Trauma Center at the Justice Resource Institute in Boston, this book offers sage advice for clinicians, teachers, and practitioners seeking trauma-sensitive yoga.

Hugh Milne, *The Heart of Listening: A Visionary Approach to Craniosacral Work* (Berkeley, CA: North Atlantic Books, 1996). A sacred map for craniosacral work, teaching us ways to feel and see the body's natural yearning for stability and alignment. A scientific and deeply personal guide for practitioners and students seeking to understand the poetry of touch.

Yoga, Meditation, and Mindfulness

Hilda Gutiérrez Baldoquín, ed. *Dharma, Color, and Culture: New Voices in Western Buddhism* (Berkeley, CA: Parallax Press, 2004). An inspiring multiracial anthology on meditation and mindfulness edited by the Western Massachusetts–based charismatic and wise Sota Zen priest, Hilda Gutiérrez Baldoquín.

T. K. V. Desikachar, *The Heart of Yoga: Developing a Personal Practice* (Rochester, VT: Inner Traditions, 1995). An intimate invitation into the profundity of yoga written by one of the most influential yogis of our time. Includes marvelous brief interpretations of the Yoga Sutras, thoughtful, deep interviews with Desikachar, comprehensive explanations of yoga fundamentals, and inspiring photographs of him and his father, Krishnamacharya.

Thich Nhat Hanh, *The Miracle of Mindfulness: A Manual of Meditation* (Boston: Beacon Press, 1976). All of Nhat Hanh's books are precious. This remains my go-to book because it has a timeless parable about eating a tangerine and tells the story about why he wrote the book after being forced into exile due to his work with both the North and South Vietnamese during the Vietnam War.

Rolf Gates and Katrina Kenison, *Meditations from the Mat: Daily Reflections on the Path of Yoga* (New York: Anchor, 2002). Written by an ex-military recovering alcoholic turned yoga teacher, this beautiful book includes 365 entries illuminating the eight limbs of yoga, drawing upon life experience, research, literature, and history for inspiration.

Sharon Salzberg, *A Heart as Wide as the World: Living with Mindfulness, Wisdom, and Compassion* (Boston: Shambhala, 1997). Written by a leading meditation teacher and writer, this book helps us know why loving kindness can bring sanity to ourselves and to the world. Salzberg's books and meditation CDs are sweet company in lonely, exciting, changing moments in our lives.

Kyczy Hawk, *Yoga and the Twelve-Step Path* (Las Vegas: Central Recovery Press, 2012). Passed on to me by Patti Mitchell, the yogi and hospice nurse who guided me as my grandmother was dying, this book offers an honest chronicling of how being "a friend of Bill's" (being in twelve-step programs) and a friend of the mat can be synergistic.

Charlotte Bell, *Mindful Yoga, Mindful Life: A Guide for Everyday Practice* (Berkeley, CA: Rodmell Press, 2007). Bell offers a delicate weaving of her personal story and teachings of the classical principles of yoga, interpreting the eight limbs as practical and gutsy ways of living.

Hari Kirin Kaur Khalsa, *Art and Yoga: Kundalini Awakening in Everyday Life* (Santa Cruz, NM: Kundalini Research Institute, 2011). This exquisitely designed book by one of Kundalini's senior teachers offers loving step-by-step guidelines for practicing yoga and art, showing the synergism between the two. The book includes a helpful chapter on dealing with difficult emotions and ways to find our infinite selves untouched by trauma.

Memoir and Autobiography

Matthew Sanford, *Waking: A Memoir of Trauma and Transcendence* (Emmaus, PA: Rodale, 2006). After a tragic car accident at age thirteen that left Sanford paralyzed from the torso down, Sanford relied upon the medical model of healing for ten years, accepting his legs as essentially dead, until finding yoga. This journey led him to become a preeminent yoga teacher for people with disabilities and everyone else seeking to understand the subtlety and sophistication of our bodies' sensations.

Stephen Cope, editor, *Will Yoga and Meditation Really Change My Life?: Personal Stories from 25 of North America's Leading Teachers* (North Adams, Massachusetts: Storey Publishing, 2003). Edited by the Director of the Kripalu Institute for Extraordinary Living, this anthology includes a marvelous set of personal essays written by leading meditators and yogis. I especially appreciate the religious, racial, and gender diversity in the book as well as the gorgeous photographs.

Mary Rose O'Reilley, *Radical Presence: Teaching as Contemplative Practice* (Portsmouth, NH: Heinemann, 1998). A slim, hilarious book by a Quaker, Buddhist, and shepherd that is about faith, teaching, and "listening like a cow."

For Veterans and Their Families

Brian Turner, *Here, Bullet* (Farmington, ME: Alice James, 2005). Winner of the prestigious Beatrice Hawley Award, Turner's poetry is the finest I have seen about the impossibility and devastation of the Iraq War as well as how writing through the body can keep vets alive.

Tim O'Brien, *The Things They Carried* (New York: Houghton Mifflin, 1990). This bone-chilling novel, based in the American war in Vietnam, taught me about how incoherent memory is the closest thing to the truth we may have in unspeakable situations, and the power of language to salvage the human spirit amid rubble and loss.

Patience H. C. Mason, *Recovering from the War: A Guide for All Veterans, Family Members, Friends and Therapists* (High Springs, FL: Patience Press, 1998). Healing for a vet is healing for a community.

The Welcome: A Healing Journey for War Veterans and Their Families (Two Shoes Productions, 2011). A documentary film for everybody who wants to welcome vets back with open arms. Brave, intimate conversations with Native American, African American, Asian American, and White Vets about isolation, despair, PTSD, as well as the power of song, poetry, contemplation, and community in healing. See www.thewelcomethemovie.com.

Poetry and Novels

While none of the books below focus on yoga directly, all teach us about the resilience of the human spirit. Given the novel's ability to describe the three-dimensionality of human life, it is no surprise that this genre is a primary source for understanding abuse and its aftermath.

Sonia Sanchez, *Morning Haiku* (Boston: Beacon Press, 2010). As one of the architects of the Black arts movement, now in her late seventies, Sanchez offers us five decades of poetry, activism, and consummate teaching. *Morning Haiku* is one of her most soulful, most meditative.

Joy Harjo, *A Map to the Next World* (New York: W. W. Norton, 2000). Written by a Muscogee poet and musician, this book helps us imagine a world where "there is no such thing as a one-way land bridge."

Dorothy Allison, *Bastard out of Carolina* (New York: Dutton, 1992). In my many readings of this novel, Allison continues to teach me about the spiritual and emotional depths of hunger and appetite, with chilling descriptions of how sexual abuse can take away girls' tears.

Edwidge Danticat, *Breath, Eyes, Memory* (New York: Vintage, 1994) is a novel by a Haitian writer about how three generations of women survive amid colonialism, war, sexual abuse, and immigration. Her lyrical language and sense of time and place make this a truly gorgeous book.

Toni Morrison, *The Bluest Eye* (New York: Holt, Rinehart and Winston, 1970). Written by the first Black woman to earn a Nobel Prize in literature, this novel teaches about what dissociation looks and feels like for girls assaulted by racism and sexual abuse.

Alice Walker, *The Color Purple* (New York: Harcourt Brace, 1982). The widely seen movie pales in comparison to this breathtaking novel about a young woman's triumph after abuse from several directions. Among other Walker books of essays and poetry, see also *Anything We Love Can Be Saved: A Writer's Activism; Absolute Trust in the Goodness of the Earth; Hard Times Require Furious Dancing,* and *Now Is the Time to Open Your Heart.*

Rafael Campo, *What the Body Told* (Durham, NC: Duke University Press, 1996), and *The Poetry of Healing: A Doctor's Education in Empathy, Identity, and Desire* (New York: W. W. Norton, 1997). Campo is a gay Cuban American physician, the William Carlos Williams of his generation, whose poetry is embodied and brave.

Trauma Theory

Cathy Caruth, editor, *Trauma: Explorations in Memory* (Baltimore: Johns Hopkins University Press, 1995). Edited by a preeminent trauma scholar and professor, this book pulls together an unprecedented range of scholars, illuminating the complexity of trauma and its aftermath.

Almost twenty years since it was first published, this remains my go-to book for understanding the psychoanalysis of trauma (and why healing is possible).

Laura van Dernoot Lipsky with Connie Burk, *Trauma Stewardship: An Everyday Guide to Caring for Self while Caring for Others* (San Francisco: Berrett-Koehler, 2009). Written by a seasoned trauma worker who understands that a daily practice of self-care is at the center of activism. Offers excellent chronicling of what burnout looks like for trauma specialists and steps to stay awake spiritually and emotionally.

Janina Fisher, "Psychoeducational Aids for Working with Psychological Trauma" (2009; available to order online at www.janinafisher.com). A concise and integrated flip chart (with graphics) that explains the dynamics of trauma, including dissociation, fight and flight, freeze and submit, signs of hyper- and hypo-arousal, and stages of trauma recovery.

Judith Herman, *Trauma and Recovery: The Aftermath of Violence—from Domestic Abuse to Political Terror* (New York: Basic Books, 1992). A foundational book on the stages of healing for sexual abuse survivors, tracing the transformation from victim to survivor.

Peter A. Levine, *Waking the Tiger: Healing Trauma* (Berkeley, CA: North Atlantic Books, 1997). Written accessibly by a biological physicist, Levine sees trauma as informative and transformative, showing how listening to the body can help people heal.

Bessel A. van der Kolk, Alexander C. McFarlane, and Lars Weisaeth, editors, *Traumatic Stress: The Effects of Overwhelming Experience on Mind, Body, and Society* (New York: Guilford Press, 1996). A seminal text on post–traumatic stress disorder edited by world-renowned trauma researcher Bessel A. van der Kolk and colleagues. Emphasizes the science and sociopolitical context of trauma as well as evidenced-based successful treatment.

Yoga Philosophy

Donna Farhi, *Bringing Yoga to Life: The Everyday Practice of Enlightened Living* (New York: Harper, 2003). Written by an internationally known yoga teacher, this book weaves yoga philosophy into understanding the long-term spiritual and emotional practice of yoga.

Alistair Shearer, translator, *The Yoga Sutras of Patanjali* (New York: Bell Tower, 1982). While there are many useful translations of Patanjali's ancient work, I particularly appreciate Shearer's nuanced and accessible analysis of the Yoga Sutras. The book's small size and its warm cover make it possible to slip into your coat pocket on a cold morning.

Stephen Cope, *The Wisdom of Yoga: A Seeker's Guide to Extraordinary Living* (New York: Bantam Books, 2006). This book walks us past delusion, aversion, and craving into places of awareness and joy through an accessible exploration of yoga philosophy. I teach this book in doctoral education classes as well as in yoga workshops. Cope is one deep thinker.

Idiosyncratic Music List

David Darling, *8-String Religion*

Juan Luis Guerra, *Colección Romantica*

India.Arie, *Acoustic Soul* and *Songversation*

Quincy Jones, *Back on the Block*

Snatam Kaur, *Grace, Liberation's Door*

Angélique Kidjo, *Black Ivory Soul*

Patti LaBelle, *Greatest Love Songs*

Ladysmith Black Mambazo, *Long Walk to Freedom*

Pablo Milanés, all of his music

Van Morrison, *Back and Top, The Healing Game,* and especially *The Philosopher's Stone*

Rahsaan Patterson, *Love in Stereo*

Silvio Rodríquez, *Cuba Classics*

Sade, *Soldier of Love*

So Amazing: An All-Star Tribute to Luther Vandross

Soulfood, *Shaman's Way*

Sweet Honey in the Rock, has been inspiring us for thirty years, multiple albums

NOTES

Acknowledgments

1. Alice Walker, "Sister Assata: This Is What American History Looks Like," Alice Walker: The Offical Website, 2013, www.alicewalkersgarden.com/2013/05/sister-assata-this-is-what-american-history-looks-like/

Introduction

1. Dissociation begins as a survival strategy when some aspect of a traumatizing event would so overwhelm the person that the mind automatically renders a part or all of the event inaccessible to the conscious self. The rage, fear, shame, or self-hate from the event is too intense to be faced at the time. Once the memory of this event is split off from the conscious self, it exerts underground pressure to emerge, which takes energy away from other parts of the self to keep it submerged. So, the defending parts may impel one to eat, or drink, or run, or be a workaholic, or abusive, or not know why we are acting as we are. The defending parts may also be self-critical—all to ward off having the experience emerge into awareness. Present experiences that may trigger old memories and emotions can feel overwhelming and confusing until reassociation can occur. This process requires healing at the level of the mind, body, and spirit, since the initial trauma split us from experiencing our most integrated selves. Healing involves being able to hold the original experience and the protective parts with understanding and compassion. This starts with feeling safe enough to do this work. Thank you to Dr. Cathy Colman for her years of clinical experience and generous teachings about dissociation and healing.

2. This was before the publication of David Emerson and Elizabeth Hopper's crucial book, *Overcoming Trauma through Yoga: Reclaiming Your Body* (Berkeley, CA: North Atlantic Books, 2011), a powerful testimony that neuroscience, Eastern-derived contemplative practices,

263

and psychotherapy are joining together now, leaving enormous clues for what healing can look like through yoga. This was also before Ana T. Forrest's *Fierce Medicine: Breakthrough Practices to Heal the Body and Ignite the Spirit* (New York: HarperOne, 2011), the first memoir written by a female yogi and trauma survivor about yoga's healing powers in the face of multiple injustices.

3. I remember that for years after I bought *The Courage to Heal: A Guide for Women Survivors of Child Sexual Abuse* (Ellen Bass and Laura Davis, New York: Perennial Library, 1988), the most I could do was keep the book close and read short sections of it in fast snatches. I was grateful to own that book and was scared by it, too.

4. Holly Near, "You Bet," *Imagine My Surprise*, Olivia Records, 1978, LP.

5. Edwidge Danticat, *Breath, Eyes, Memory* (New York: Vintage, 1994), 25.

6. In some instances throughtout this book, the people whose stories are included chose pseudonyms to protect their own and others' privacy.

7. "Living in the body" is a felt sense of understanding your body as your own: this includes being able to find and experience your breath, pulse, and movement (dancing, walking, singing, whispering *namaste*); feeling safe and alive in your body, including its pleasures; being able to stay in your body even when difficult emotions or injuries make it tempting to numb out or seek unhelpful distractions; feeling your bodily parameters (where you stop and another person starts); being conscious of your toes, fingers, eyes, elbows, cheeks, stomach, and heart, as well as the (hopefully loving) energy you send into the world; and wanting to honor your body as a temple (since it is).

8. Throughout the text, I use the English translation of yoga terms followed by the term in Sanskrit. I include both languages out of respect for yoga's origins and because the Sanskrit terms embody a cadence that resonates with the deep meaning of the poses—i.e. you can feel the energy of the pose in the sounds of the Sanskrit words.

9. The first limb, the yamas, includes five ethical principles, also called the laws of life: nonviolence *(ahimsa),* truthfulness *(satya),* integrity *(asteya),* sexual accountability *(brahmacharya),* and nonattachment *(aparigraha).* The second limb, the niyamas, includes five ethical observances, or rules for living: simplicity *(sauca),* contentment *(santosa),* purification *(tapas),* self-study, refinement *(svadhyaya)* and devotion *(isvara-pranidhana).* For an excellent translation of the Yoga Sutras, see Alistair Shearer, trans., *The Yoga Sutras of Patanjali* (New York: Bell Tower, 1982).

Part I. Deeper than Words: Finding the Mat

1. For descriptions of these yoga traditions, see Appendix III. Shakti yoga dance was created by dancer, choreographer, yogi, and Wellesley College instructor Samantha Cameron. Samantha choreographs intricate dances with yoga postures to create original pieces that yoga practitioners then perform together. For more about Shakti dancing, see http://dailybreathjournal.com.

2. Adrienne Rich, "Prospective Immigrants Please Note," *The Fact of a Doorframe: Poems Selected and New 1950–1984* (New York: Norton, 1984), 51–52.

3. Amy Weintraub, *Yoga for Depression: A Compassionate Guide to Relieve Suffering through Yoga* (New York: Random House, 2004), 201.

4. Becky Thompson, *A Hunger So Wide and So Deep: A Multiracial View of Woman's Eating Problems* (Minneapolis: University of Minnesota Press, 1994).

5. Donna Farhi, *Bringing Yoga to Life: The Everyday Practice of Enlightened Living* (New York: Harper, 2003), 20.

6. Daniel Siegel, "Interpersonal Neurobiology of Trauma Resolution," Trauma and Neuroscience Conference, Lesley University, Cambridge, MA, July 7, 2011. Keynote lecture.

7. Hugh Milne, *The Heart of Listening: A Visionary Approach to Craniosacral Work* (Berkeley, CA: North Atlantic Books, 1996), 80.

8. Thank you to yogi Cat Kabira for her wisdom in using the word *portal* as a way to describe early access to seeing energy and for her teachings on the energetics of yoga.

9. Pam Houston praise for Tempest Williams, *When Women Were Birds: Fifty-Four Variations on Voice* (New York: Farrar, Straus and Giroux, 2012), back cover.

10. David Read Johnson, "Using Play as an Exposure Therapy for Traumatized Children," Trauma and Neuroscience Conference, Lesley University, Cambridge, MA, July 8, 2011.

11. Chris Newbound, "Yoga's Impact on Post-Traumatic Stress Disorder," *Kripalu* (2010–2011), 5.

12. Ibid., 3.

13. Ibid., 5.

14. Brian Turner, *Here, Bullet* (Farmington, ME: Alice James, 2005).

15. Ibid., 45.

16. Shearer, *Yoga Sutras,* 90 (Sutra I.1–2).

17. Retrospectively, she also saw the metaphorical significance of asthma. As a child growing up in a family where alcoholism and deferred dreams were not verbalized but ever present, she took on the family's grief. As Ana T. Forrest explains, "Grief commonly shows up in the lungs as congestion, asthma, or other forms of entrapment. . . . You can drown in your own grief when those areas aren't in motion" (*Fierce Medicine,* 51).

18. Patricia Walden, "Moving from Darkness into Light," in *Will Yoga and Meditation Really Change My Life?: Personal Stories from 25 of North America's Leading Teachers,* ed. Stephen Cope (North Adams, MA: Storey Publishing, 2003), 89–90.

19. Ibid., 90.

20. Ibid., 90.

21. Ibid., 91–92.

22. Matthew Sanford, *Waking: A Memoir of Trauma and Transcendence* (Emmaus, PA: Rodale, 2006), 192–93.

23. Ibid., 192.

24. Ibid., 216.

25. Ibid.

26. Joy Harjo, *A Map to the Next World* (New York: W. W. Norton, 2000), 17.

27. Konda Mason, "Nonviolent Activism with Wisdom," in *Yoga and Meditation,* ed. Stephen Cope (North Adams, MA: Storey Publishing, 2003), 111.

28. Ibid., 112.

29. Ibid., 113.

30. Sonia Sanchez, "10 Haiku," *Morning Haiku* (Boston: Beacon Press, 2010), 17.

31. For more about Wyoma, including her teaching of African dance and holistic therapy, see her video *African American Healing Dance* (Sounds True, 1998), DVD, and www.wyomadance.com.

32. For more about Anna Dunwell, her yoga studio, Soul Sanctuary, and her teaching, see www.annadunwell.com.

33. Breath of joy is a three-part inhalation as you fling your arms toward the sky, to your side, and over your head again before cascading your arms

to the ground with a big exhale. This synchronized movement, which is typically done ten or more times, promises bursts of prana followed by happy relaxation. The collective circle poses include tree to forest (vrksasana), petal pose *(navasana)*, and balancing stick *(tuladandasana)*.

34. Thank you to Peg McAdam for first introducing me to how to transform tree pose (vrksasana) into a forest.

Part II. Like Dragonflies: What Makes Trauma Survivors Special

1. Martín Espada, *Imagine the Angels of Bread* (New York: Norton, 1996), 93.

2. Akasha Gloria Hull, *Soul Talk: The New Spirituality of African American Women* (Rochester, VT: Inner Traditions, 2001), 142.

3. Gloria Anzaldúa, "La Prieta," in *This Bridge Called My Back: Writings by Radical Women of Color,* eds. Cherríe Moraga and Gloria Anzaldúa (New York: Kitchen Table Women of Color Press, 1983), 208.

4. Anzaldúa writes that "left-handed guardians . . . are busy beavers (and like them also an endangered species). . . . Wherever we are we make sure there are several entrances and exits. . . . We work hard at building community. Our strength lies in shifting perspectives, in our capacity to shift, in our 'seeing through' the membrane of the past superimposed on the present, in looking at our shadows and dealing with them." Gloria Anzaldúa, "Haciendo Caras, Una Entrada," in *Making Face, Making Soul/ Haciendo Caras: Creative and Critical Perspectives by Women of Color,* ed. Gloria Anzaldúa (San Francisco: Aunt Lute, 1990), xxvi–xxvii. Living with this consciousness births a kind of "psychic restlessness," about the world as it is, a knowing that what *is* does not have to be. Psychic restlessness comes from an awareness that injustices are not inevitable, that people are often asked to rally against themselves, to follow rules that are not in their interests. Many trauma survivors live with this "psychic restlessness"—an insecurity, a vague discomfort, a questioning spirit—that comes from having seen the world from its underbelly. Gloria Anzaldúa, "La Conciencia de la Mestiza: Toward a New Consciousness" (377–89) in *Making Face, Making Soul/ Haciendo Caras,* 377.

5. Milne, *Heart of Listening,* 73–74.

6. Bonnie Burstow, "Toward a Radical Understanding of Trauma and Trauma Work," *Violence Against Women* 9: 11 (November 2003), 1298.

7. Rolf Gates and Katrina Kenison, *Meditations from the Mat: Daily Reflections on the Path of Yoga* (New York: Anchor, 2002), 21–22.

8. The tango class, taught by Danny Trenner, was held at Dance New England, a crazy fun camp in Freedom, New Hampshire, open to everyone who loves to dance late into the night, make pancakes in the morning, practice AcroYoga at lunch, and Thai massage to the moon.

9. In Spanish, *salida* means "exit," which, in tango, means a way out of the anticipation before the dance and into the dance itself, the transition from the given world into the vortex of mystery and movement.

10. Donna Farhi (*Bringing Yoga to Life*, 138) writes, "Within the natural mind lives a domain of information that we cannot find through the normal channels of our habitual, rational mind."

11. Stephen Cope, *The Wisdom of Yoga: A Seeker's Guide to Extraordinary Living* (New York: Bantam Books, 2006), 31.

12. Farhi, *Bringing Yoga to Life*, 138.

13. Pema Chödrön, *When Things Fall Apart: Heart Advice for Difficult Times* (Boston: Shambhala, 1997), 53–59.

14. Akasha Gloria Hull, *Soul Talk: The New Spirituality of African American Women* (Rochester, VT: Inner Traditions, 2001), 142.

15. Furious Flower Poetry Center tribute to the poet, playwright, and activist Sonia Sanchez. James Madison University, June 20–24, 2011.

16. T. K. V. Desikachar, *The Heart of Yoga: Developing a Personal Practice* (Rochester, VT: Inner Traditions, 1995), 88.

17. Thompson, *Hunger So Wide.*

18. Joy Harjo, "Bird," *In Mad Love and War* (Middletown, CT: Wesleyan University Press, 1990), 21.

19. Desikachar, *Heart of Yoga,* 55.

20. Ibid., 87.

21. Tutu explains the meaning of ubuntu with the African proverb, "A person is a person through other persons." Our essence, as people, comes from our belonging. Desmond Tutu, *No Future without Forgiveness* (New York: Doubleday, 1999), 31.

22. Desikachar, *Heart of Yoga,* 86.

23. I call the circumstances "extraordinary" even though many traumas—child abuse; physical, sexual, and mental abuse; police brutality—are common. Regardless of how common, the experience of it in our bodies is still extraordinary, flooding the senses, leaving a blank spot in memory, shocking us to the point of freezing.

24. William J. Broad, *The Science of Yoga: The Risks and the Rewards* (New York: Simon and Schuster, 2012), 90.

25. Janina Fisher, "Psychoeducational Aids for Working with Psychological Trauma," 2009. Available to order online, www.janinafisher.com.

26. Linda Hogan, *Dwellings: A Spiritual History of the Living World* (New York: Simon & Schuster, 1995), 26.

27. Ibid., 27.

28. Ibid., 26.

29. Ibid., 25.

30. Ibid., 26.

31. Ibid., 26.

Part III. Hide and Seek: The Circuitous Path of Healing

1. Pema Chödrön and Alice Walker, *In Conversation: On the Meaning of Suffering and the Mystery of Joy* (Boulder, CO: Sounds True, 1999), audio tape.

2. Mary Rose O'Reilley, *The Barn at the End of the World: The Apprenticeship of a Quaker, Buddhist Shepherd* (Minneapolis: Milkweed Editions, 2000).

3. A midwife friend, Carol Leonard, says that when a woman has thirteen cycles in a row without her period, then the process is complete. In the land of midwifery, this is seen as an ending—of the possibility of making new life—and a beginning, of the next cycle.

4. Cope, *Wisdom of Yoga*, 115.

5. The sequence of poses focuses on opening the heart, an approach based on the understanding that lupus begins from an energetic block in the heart.

6. Personal conversation with John Brown, yoga practitioner. (John is also profiled in "Like a Homily," pages 50–52.)

7. The clarifications about desire are all paraphrased from a lecture given by Feldman at the Insight Meditation Center in Barre, Massachusetts, as explained by Ginger Norwood. See also Christina Feldman, *Compassion: Listening to the Cries of the World* (Berkeley, CA: Rodmell Press, 2005).

8. Cope, *Wisdom of Yoga*, 221.

9. Milne, *Heart of Listening*, 81.

10. Shearer, *Yoga Sutras,* 92 (Sutra I.14).

11. Ibid.

12. Geri Larkin, *Stumbling toward Enlightenment* (Berkeley, CA: Celestial Arts, 2009), 217.

13. India.Arie, "Beautiful Flower," *Testimony: Vol. 2, Love & Politics* (Universal, 2007), Audio CD.

14. Pema Chödrön, *No Time to Lose: A Timely Guide to the Way of the Bodhisattva* (Boston: Shambhala, 2005).

15. Eknath Easwaran, *Meditation* (Tomales, CA: Nilgiri Press, 1971), 190.

16. Shearer, *Yoga Sutras,* 110 (Sutra II.46).

17. Larkin, *Stumbling Toward Enlightenment,* 41.

18. Ibid., 40.

19. Stephen Cope, "The Yoga Sutra Course," Kripalu Center for Yoga and Health, Stockbridge, MA, April 16–18, 2011.

20. Tara Brach, *Radical Acceptance: Embracing Your Life with the Heart of a Buddha* (New York: Bantam Books, 2003), 103.

21. Sanchez, *Morning Haiku,* preface page.

22. Shearer, *Yoga Sutras,* 90 (Sutra I.3).

Part IV. The Color of Rothko's Blue: Long-Term Wholeness

1. Farhi, *Bringing Yoga to Life,* 145.

2. Richard Miller, "The Search for Oneness," in Cope, *Yoga and Meditation,* 139.

3. Doug Keller, "Kundalini, Chakras, Tantra, and Guided Meditation," public talk, Arlington Center, MA, October 9, 2011.

4. Devadas Day, Kripalu Center for Yoga and Health, Stockbridge, MA, August 6, 2011. This teacher, with sweet, shy eyes and long gray hair, opens his "rigorous vinyasa" practices with short dharma talks that are so smart, distilled, and wise that I find myself taking notes, even as I try to do the postures.

5. Furious Flower Poetry Center tribute to the poet, playwright, and activist Sonia Sanchez, James Madison University, June 20–24, 2011.

6. Becky Thompson, *Mothering without a Compass: White Mother's Love, Black Son's Courage* (Minneapolis: University of Minnesota, 2000).

7. Another time I experienced this channeling was when my friend and fellow yoga practitioner Diane Harriford and I wrote about the unleashing of historical memory in the aftermath of Hurricane Katrina. For details about this process, see Diane Harriford and Becky Thompson, *When the Center Is on Fire: Passionate Social Theory for Our Times* (Austin: University of Texas Press, 2008).

8. Hari Kirin Kaur Khalsa, *Art and Yoga: Kundalini Awakening in Everyday Life* (Santa Cruz, NM: Kundalini Research Institute, 2011).

9. Shearer, *Yoga Sutras,* 69.

10. Peg McAdam, personal conversation, July 23, 2011.

11. Barbara Stoler Miller, *Yoga: Discipline of Freedom: The Yoga Sutra Attributed to Patanjali* (New York: Bantam Books, 1998), 61.

12. Farhi, *Bringing Yoga to Life,* 21.

13. Recorded by Sweet Honey in the Rock as "Alla Tha's All Right, but," *Breaths* (Flying Fish Records, 1980). Written by June Jordan, "Alla Tha's All Right, but," *Directed by Desire: The Collected Poems of June Jordan* (Port Townsend, WA: Copper Canyon Press, 2005), 285.

14. Rama Berch, "I Always Belonged to God," in Cope, *Yoga and Meditation,* 237–38.

15. Audre Lorde, *Sister Outsider: Essays and Speeches* (Freedom, CA: Crossing Press, 1984), 53–59.

16. Shearer, *Yoga Sutras,* 60–61.

17. Hozan Alan Senauke, "On Race and Buddhism," in *Making the Invisible Visible: Healing Racism in Our Buddhist Communities,* Larry Yang, ed., http://insightpv.org/Storage/Making%20the%20Invisible%20Visible-11.pdf.

18. Two days after she gave me my instructions, when we were sitting quietly, I asked her if she could describe the space she had been going into in the last months. She said, "It is a longing to stay there," her answer revealing a place that she was not fearing, in fact had been contacting and wanting to stay.

19. Only later, after she passed, did I learn from a hospice nurse that during the active part of the dying process, in rare instances of congestive heart failure, the lungs will release material long held, as is similar to the release of other bodily fluids right before death. At the time, a memory from a yoga anatomy class about how the diaphragm breathes the lungs from a space below the lungs helped me accompany her through this difficult time.

20. I recall a yogi training in Colorado where the instructors flapped mats, made inane conversation, and flashed the lights on and off during a practice to teach us to stay quiet and within ourselves during a practice.

21. Shearer, *Yoga Sutras,* 111–12 (Sutra II.49–55).

22. Charlotte Bell, *Mindful Yoga, Mindful Life: A Guide for Everyday Practice* (Berkeley, CA: Rodmell Press, 2007), 160.

Part V. In the Shadow of the Temple: The Special Work of Teachers

1. Kahlil Gibran, *The Prophet* (New York: Alfred A. Knopf, 2000), 62.

2. Shearer, *Yoga Sutras,* 96 (Sutra I.37).

3. Desikachar, *Heart of Yoga,* 116.

4. Bessel A. van der Kolk and Dana Moore, "Frontiers of Trauma Treatment," Kripalu Center for Yoga and Health, Stockbridge, MA, October 28–30, 2011.

5. For a fascinating account of the complexity and deep contradictions of Bikram Choudhury's life, see Benjamin Lorr, *Hell-Bent: Obsession, Pain, and the Search for Something Like Transcendence in Competitive Yoga* (New York: St. Martins, 2012).

6. Forrest, *Fierce Medicine,* 1.

7. Ibid., 4.

8. Ibid., 137.

9. Ibid., 133.

10. As one of her certified teachers wrote to me, "My experience is that Ana's commitment to train women to be so strong and fierce is an expression of her own healing. No one every taught me those things. The punch line is that she uses teacher training to help survivors (a huge percentage of whom come to her) to find their bodies and voices and fight for their lives." Karuna O'Donnell, personal correspondence, February 12, 2013.

11. Forrest, *Fierce Medicine,* 122.

12. As Forrest writes, "although I studied Yoga with B. K. S. Iyengar himself, the most important lesson I learned from him was to disobey the dictator if you don't find a man's character congruent with his teachings" (Forrest, *Fierce Medicine,* 2).

13. Wendy Rose, "The Great Pretenders: Further Reflections on Whiteshamanism," in *The State of Native America: Genocide, Colonization, and*

Resistance, ed. M. Annette Jaimes (Boston: South End Press, 1992), 403–22.

14. Forrest, *Fierce Medicine,* 2.

15. Ibid., 171.

16. Unlike many yogis, Max bucks the contemporary tendency to consider yoga a spiritual rather than a religious practice. She reasons that yoga qualifies as a religion since it is practiced in a communal way, has its own ethical system, includes devotional rituals, and has specific locations for gathering and connection. Her evolving perspective reflects her research in comparative religions and her own path as a yogi, in particular her transformation from treating yoga as an intense physical practice to recognizing its spiritual dimensions.

17. Kyczy Hawk, *Yoga and the Twelve-Step Path* (Las Vegas: Central Recovery Press, 2012), x.

18. Ibid., 98. For more about Nikki Myers and her innovative grassroots program, see www.y12sr.com. See also the twice-annual Yoga, Meditation and Recovery Conference held at various locations in the United States.

19. Hawk, *Yoga and the Twelve-Step Path,* 99.

20. Becky Thompson, "You Know Survivors, We," *Zero Is the Whole I Fall into at Night* (Charlotte, NC: Main Street Rag, 2011), 29.

21. For more on the power of witnessing, see Cathy Caruth, ed., *Trauma: Explorations in Memory* (Baltimore: Johns Hopkins University Press, 1995). Caruth's volume shows us that trauma causes "the inability to fully witness the event as it occurs, or the ability to witness the event fully only at the cost of witnessing oneself" (7). As a consequence, witnessing the story of those who have been traumatized is crucial to help release the memory's hold. Such witnessing requires deep listening, since traumatic memory is unlike that of ordinary memory; it is nonlinear, fragmented. Dissociation begins as a means of psychic protection; it also provides essential data for healing.

22. June Jordan, "Poem for South African Women," *Directed by Desire: The Collected Poems of June Jordan* (Port Townsend, WA: Copper Canyon Press, 2005), 279.

23. Desikachar, *Heart of Yoga,* 53.

24. Weintraub, *Yoga for Depression,* 202.

25. Chris Newbound, "Kripalu's Institute for Extraordinary Living Launches a Pioneering Study to Determine Yoga's Effect on Soldiers and Veterans Suffering from PTSD." *Kripalu* (2010–2011), 3–7.

26. Weintraub, *Yoga for Depression*, 202.

27. Wynton Marsalis, "Happy Birthday Lincoln Center: A New York Treasure for 50 Years." *The New York Times Magazine*, May 10, 2009, 26F.

28. David Read Johnson, "Using Play as an Exposure Therapy for Traumatized Children," Trauma and Neuroscience Conference, Lesley University, July 8, 2011.

29. Sweet Honey in the Rock, "Dream Variations," *Sweet Honey in the Rock* (Flying Fish, 1976).

30. Peg Mulqueen, "Those Who Can, Teach," *Yoga Journal* (October 2011), 80–85.

Part VI. "Love Calls Us to the Things of This World": Yoga and Activism

1. Cope, *Wisdom of Yoga*, xxvi.

2. Rosa Zubizarreta, "Personal Statement," in Yang, *Making the Invisible Visible*, 31.

3. Sylvia Boorstein, "I Got Kinder," in Cope, *Yoga and Meditation*, 26.

4. Richard Wilber, "Love Calls Us to the Things of this World," *New and Collected Poems* (New York: Harcourt, 1988), 233–34. This poem was first introduced to me by Mary Rose O'Reilley in her book *Radical Presence: Teaching as Contemplative Practice* (Portsmouth, NH: Heinemann, 1998).

5. Robin D. G. Kelley, *Freedom Dreams: The Black Radical Imagination* (Boston: Beacon Press, 2002), 2–3.

6. Ibid., 1.

7. Hilda Gutiérrez Baldoquín, "Don't Waste Time," in *Dharma, Color, and Culture: New Voices in Western Buddhism*, ed. Hilda Gutiérrez Baldoquín (Berkeley, CA: Parallax Press, 2004), 182.

8. Larkin, *Stumbling Toward Enlightenment*, 13.

9. Jarvis Jay Masters, *Finding Freedom: Writings from Death Row* (Junction City, CA: Padma Publishing, 1997), 169–73.

10. Ibid., 173.

11. Alice Walker, "Edwidge Danticat, the Quiet Stream," Facebook, January 23, 2010.

12. Mason, "Nonviolent Activism," *Yoga and Meditation,* 113.

13. Ginger Norwood and Ouyporn Khuankaew are cofounders of the International Women's Partnership for Peace and Justice in Thailand: http://womenforpeaceandjustice.org.

14. Daniel Siegel, "Interpersonal Neurobiology of Trauma Resolution," Trauma and Neuroscience Conference, Lesley University, July 7, 2011, keynote lecture. Siegel gave a graphic example of the difference between current versus infinite possibilities by explaining that while current possibilities might lead him to describe himself as "a doctor who studies the brain who is from California," an awareness of infinite possibilities allows him to describe himself relationally: "we are on common ground, my open plane is your open plane. You are me and I am you." Both the current possibilities and infinite possibilities are true; one clearly making way for a relationality and expansiveness that the first social address precludes.

15. Sanchez, "Haiku Poem: 1 Year after 9/11," *Morning Haiku,* 97.

16. Suheir Hammad, "First Writing Since," in *Trauma at Home: After 9/11,* ed. Judith Greenberg (Lincoln, NE: University of Nebraska Press, 2003), 139.

17. Moustafa Bayoumi, *How Does It Feel to Be a Problem?* (New York: Penguin, 2008), cited in Harriford and Thompson *When the Center Is on Fire,* 90.

18. Shearer, *Yoga Sutras,* 64–65.

19. Kai Erikson, "Notes on Trauma and Community," in Caruth, *Trauma: Explorations in Memory,* 187.

20. The Harriet Tubman House, named after the African American abolitionist who escaped slavery and helped to free hundreds of other slaves, is a community center in a historically multiracial neighborhood in Boston.

21. Audre Lorde, *The Cancer Journals* (Argyle, NY: Spinsters Ink, 1980).

22. Thompson, "Naptime in the Basement," *Zero Is the Whole,* 18.

23. Lorde, *Sister Outsider,* 53–59.

24. Cope, *Wisdom of Yoga,* 84.

25. Cited in Gates and Kenison, *Meditations from the Mat,* 398.

26. Jack Kornfield, *After the Ecstasy, the Laundry: How the Heart Grows Wise on the Spiritual Path* (New York: Bantam Books, 2000).

27. Danna Faulds, "Allow," *Go In and In: Poems from the Heart of Yoga* (Greenville, VA: Peaceable Kingdom Books, 2002), 25.

28. Chödrön and Walker, *In Conversation.*

29. White Bison, *The Red Road to Wellbriety: In the Native American Way* (Colorado Springs, CO: White Bison, 2002), Appendix 2.

30. Ibid.

31. Eve Ensler, "Suddenly, My Body," Ted Talks, www.ted.com/talks/eve_ensler.html.

32. Charles Johnston, *The Yoga Sutras of Patanjali: The Book of the Spiritual Man* (1912; repr. Teddington, UK: The Echo Library, 2006), 24–25.

33. Edwidge Danticat, *Breath, Eyes, Memory* (New York: Vintage, 1994), 25.

34. Ibid., 47.

Appendix III: Finding the Yoga That Works for You

1. My emphasis on self-reflection partly comes from understanding that teaching yoga does not, in itself, protect people from abusing their power, from causing harm to people. The history of yoga leaders who have been unethical and/or abusive has required many to separate the individual leaders from the gifts they have offered the world. This reality reminds us of our own need to practice ahimsa (nonviolence), satya (honesty), and brahmacharya (sexual responsibility) as well as compassion and forgiveness.

2. Thank you to so many people who brainstormed with me about this appendix, with such generosity, including: Hari Kirin Kaur Khalsa (Kundalini); David Emerson (Trauma-Sensitive Yoga); Liz Owen (Iyengar); Karuna O'Donnell (Forrest); Joshua Summers (Yin Yoga); David Schouela (Restorative); Diane Gardner Ducharme (Bikram); and Amy Weintraub (LifeForce Yoga).

3. To my knowledge, Ana T. Forrest and Nikki Myers (see the Y12SR entry) are the first two women who have created nationally known contemporary yoga approaches who also openly identify as trauma survivors.

4. The Kripalu Center for Yoga and Health, in western Massachusetts, a major location for teaching training and yoga instruction, is also on the cutting edge of sponsoring yoga and trauma research. The Center also hosts highly respected teachers and programs year-round for people interested in yoga, health, and healing. There are some scholarships and work-exchange programs available.

5. For a useful book on the types of yoga, see Meagan McCrary, *Pick Your Yoga Practice: Exploring and Understanding Different Styles of Yoga* (Novato, CA: New World Library, 2013). See also Jennifer Cook, "Not All Yoga Is Created Equal." *Yoga Journal* (February 24, 2010), www.yoga-journal.com/basics/165.

BIBLIOGRAPHY

Allison, Dorothy. *Bastard out of Carolina*. New York: Dutton, 1992.

Anzaldúa, Gloria. "La Prieta." In *This Bridge Called My Back: Writings by Radical Women of Color*, edited by Cherríe Moraga and Gloria Anzaldúa. New York: Kitchen Table Women of Color Press, 1983.

———, ed. *Making Face, Making Soul/Haciendo Caras: Creative and Critical Perspectives by Women of Color*. San Francisco: Aunt Lute, 1990.

Baldoquín, Hilda Gutiérrez, ed. *Dharma, Color, and Culture: New Voices in Western Buddhism*. Berkeley, CA: Parallax Press, 2004.

Bass, Ellen, and Laura Davis. *The Courage to Heal: A Guide for Women Survivors of Child Sexual Abuse*. New York: Perennial Library, 1988.

Bayoumi, Moustafa. *How Does It Feel to Be a Problem?: Being Young and Arab in American*. New York: Penguin, 2008.

Bell, Charlotte. *Mindful Yoga, Mindful Life: A Guide for Everyday Practice*. Berkeley, CA: Rodmell Press, 2007.

Berch, Rama. "I Always Belonged to God." In *Will Yoga and Meditation Really Change My Life?: Personal Stories from 25 of North America's Leading Teachers*, edited by Stephen Cope, 232–39. North Adams, MA: Storey Publishing, 2003.

Boorstein, Sylvia. "I Got Kinder," in Cope, *Yoga and Meditation*, 12–27.

Brach, Tara. *Radical Acceptance: Embracing Your Life with the Heart of a Buddha*. New York: Bantam Books, 2003.

Broad, William J. *The Science of Yoga: The Risks and the Rewards*. New York: Simon and Schuster, 2012.

Burstow, Bonnie. "Toward a Radical Understanding of Trauma and Trauma Work." *Violence Against Women* 9:11 (November 2003).

Campo, Rafael. *The Poetry of Healing: A Doctor's Education in Empathy, Identity, and Desire*. New York: W. W. Norton, 1997.

———. *What the Body Told*. Durham, NC: Duke University Press, 1996.

Caruth, Cathy, ed. *Trauma: Explorations in Memory*. Baltimore: Johns Hopkins University Press, 1995.

Chödrön, Pema. *When Things Fall Apart: Heart Advice for Difficult Times*. Boston: Shambhala, 1997.

Chödrön, Pema, and Alice Walker. *In Conversation: On the Meaning of Suffering and the Mystery of Joy*. Boulder, CO: Sounds True, 1999. Audio tape.

Cook, Jennifer. "Not All Yoga Is Created Equal." *Yoga Journal* (February 24, 2010), www.yogajournal.com/basics/165.

Cope, Stephen, ed. *Will Yoga and Meditation Really Change My Life?: Personal Stories from 25 of North America's Leading Teachers*. North Adams, MA: Storey Publishing, 2003.

———. *The Wisdom of Yoga: A Seeker's Guide to Extraordinary Living*. New York: Bantam Books, 2006.

Danticat, Edwidge. *Breath, Eyes, Memory*. New York: Vintage, 1994.

DeSalvo, Louise. *Writing as a Way of Healing: How Telling Our Stories Transforms Our Lives*. New York: HarperOne, 1999.

Desikachar, T. K. V. *The Heart of Yoga: Developing a Personal Practice*. Rochester, VT: Inner Traditions, 1995.

Emerson, David, and Elizabeth Hopper. *Overcoming Trauma through Yoga: Reclaiming Your Body*. Berkeley, CA: North Atlantic Books, 2011.

Ensler, Eve. "Suddenly, My Body." Ted Talks, www.ted.com/talks/eve_ensler.html.

Espada, Martín. *Imagine the Angels of Bread: Poems*. New York: Norton, 1996.

Erikson, Kai. "Notes on Trauma and Community." In Caruth, *Trauma*, 183–99.

Farhi, Donna. *Bringing Yoga to Life: The Everyday Practice of Enlightened Living*. New York: Harper, 2003.

Faulds, Donna. *Go In and In: Poems from the Heart of Yoga*. Greenville, VA: Peaceable Kingdom Books, 2002.

Feldman, Christina. *Compassion: Listening to the Cries of the World*. Berkeley, CA: Rodmell Press, 2005.

Forrest, Ana T. *Fierce Medicine: Breakthrough Practices to Heal the Body and Ignite the Spirit*. New York: HarperOne, 2011.

Gates, Rolf, and Katrina Kenison. *Meditations from the Mat: Daily Reflections on the Path of Yoga*. New York: Anchor, 2002.

Gibran, Kahlil. *The Prophet.* New York: Alfred A. Knopf, 2000.

Hammad, Suheir. "First Writing Since." In *Trauma at Home: After 9/11*, edited by Judith Greenberg, 139–46. Lincoln, NE: University of Nebraska Press, 2003.

Harjo, Joy. *In Mad Love and War.* Middletown, CT: Wesleyan University Press, 1990.

———. *A Map to the Next World: Poetry and Tales.* New York: W. W. Norton, 2000.

Hawk, Kyczy. *Yoga and the Twelve-Step Path.* Las Vegas: Central Recovery Press, 2012.

Hogan, Linda. *Dwellings: A Spiritual History of the Living World.* New York: Simon & Schuster, 1995.

hooks, bell. *Sisters of the Yam: Black Women and Self-Recovery.* Boston: South End Press, 1993.

Herman, Judith. *Trauma and Recovery: The Aftermath of Violence—from Domestic Abuse to Political Terror.* New York: Basic Books, 1992.

Hull, Akasha Gloria. *Soul Talk: The New Spirituality of African American Women.* Rochester, VT: Inner Traditions, 2001.

Johnston, Charles. *The Yoga Sutras of Patanjali: The Book of the Spiritual Man.* 1912; repr. Teddington, UK: The Echo Library, 2006.

Jordan, June. *Directed by Desire: The Collected Poems of June Jordan.* Port Townsend, WA: Copper Canyon Press, 2005.

Kelley, Robin D. G. *Freedom Dreams: The Black Radical Imagination.* Boston: Beacon Press, 2002.

Khalsa, Hari Kirin Kaur. *Art and Yoga: Kundalini Awakening in Everyday Life.* Santa Cruz, NM: Kundalini Research Institute, 2011.

Kornfield, Jack. *After the Ecstasy, the Laundry: How the Heart Grows Wise on the Spiritual Path.* New York: Bantam Books, 2000.

Larkin, Geri. *Stumbling toward Enlightenment.* Berkeley, CA: Celestial Arts, 2009.

Levine, Peter A. *Waking the Tiger: Healing Trauma.* Berkeley, CA: North Atlantic Books, 1997.

Lorde, Audre. *The Cancer Journals.* Argyle, NY: Spinsters Ink, 1980.

———. *Sister Outsider: Essays and Speeches.* Freedom, CA: Crossing Press, 1984.

Lorr, Benjamin. *Hell-Bent: Obsession, Pain, and the Search for Something Like Transcendence in Competitive Yoga*. New York: St. Martins, 2012.

Mason, Konda. "Nonviolent Activism with Wisdom." In Cope, *Yoga and Meditation*, 108–13.

Mason, Patience H. C. *Recovering from the War: A Guide for All Veterans, Family Members, Friends and Therapists*. High Springs, FL: Patience Press, 1998.

Masters, Jarvis Jay. *Finding Freedom: Writings from Death Row*. Junction City, CA: Padma Publishing, 1997.

McCrary, Meagan. *Pick Your Yoga Practice: Exploring and Understanding Different Styles of Yoga*. Novato, CA: New World Library, 2013.

Miller, Barbara Stoler. *Yoga: Discipline of Freedom: The Yoga Sutra Attributed to Patanjali*. New York: Bantam Books, 1998.

Miller, Richard. "The Search for Oneness." In Cope, *Yoga and Meditation*, 136–49.

Milne, Hugh. *The Heart of Listening: A Visionary Guide to Craniosacral Work*. Berkeley, CA: North Atlantic Books, 1996.

Moraga, Cherríe, and Gloria Anzaldúa, eds. *This Bridge Called My Back: Writings by Radical Women of Color*. New York: Kitchen Table Women of Color Press, 1983.

Morrison, Toni. *The Bluest Eye*. New York: Holt, Rinehart and Winston, 1970.

Mulqueen, Peg. "Those Who Can, Teach." *Yoga Journal* (October 2011), 80–85.

Newbound, Chris. "Kripalu's Institute for Extraordinary Living Launches a Pioneering Study to Determine Yoga's Effect on Soldiers and Veterans S uffering from PTSD." *Kripalu* (2010–2011), 3–7.

———. "Yoga's Impact on Post-Traumatic Stress Disorder." *Kripalu* (2010–2011).

Nhat Hanh, Thich. *The Miracle of Mindfulness: A Manual of Meditation*. Boston: Beacon Press, 1976.

O'Brien, Tim. *The Things They Carried*. New York: Houghton Mifflin, 1990.

O'Reilley, Mary Rose. *The Barn at the End of the World: The Apprenticeship of a Quaker, Buddhist Shepherd*. Minneapolis: Milkweed Editions, 2000.

———. *Radical Presence: Teaching as Contemplative Practice*. Portsmouth, NH: Heinemann, 1998.

Rich, Adrienne. *The Fact of a Doorframe: Poems Selected and New 1950–1984.* New York: Norton, 1984.

Rose, Wendy. "The Great Pretenders: Further Reflections on Whiteshamanism." In *The State of Native America: Genocide, Colonization, and Resistance,* edited by M. Annette Jaimes, 403–22. Boston: South End Press, 1992.

Sanchez, Sonia. *Morning Haiku.* Boston: Beacon Press, 2010.

Sanford, Matthew. *Waking: A Memoir of Trauma and Transcendence.* Emmaus, PA: Rodale, 2006.

Salzberg, Sharon. *A Heart as Wide as the World: Living with Mindfulness, Wisdom, and Compassion.* Boston: Shambhala, 1997.

Senauke, Hozan Alan. "On Race and Buddhism." In *Making the Invisible Visible: Healing Racism in Our Buddhist Communities,* Larry Yang, ed., 41–45, http://larryyang.org/images/MTIV,_3_ed.pdf.

Shearer, Alistair, trans. *The Yoga Sutras of Patanjali.* New York: Bell Tower, 1982.

Thompson, Becky. *A Hunger So Wide and So Deep: Eating Problems and Recovery from a Multiracial Perspective.* Minneapolis: University of Minnesota Press, 1994.

———. *Mothering without a Compass: White Mother's Love, Black Son's Courage.* Minneapolis: University of Minnesota, 2000.

———. *When the Center Is on Fire: Passionate Social Theory for Our Times.* Austin: University of Texas Press, 2008.

———. *Zero Is the Whole I Fall into at Night.* Charlotte, NC: Main Street Rag, 2011.

Turner, Brian. *Here, Bullet.* Farmington, ME: Alice James, 2005.

Tutu, Desmond. *No Future without Forgiveness.* New York: Doubleday, 1999.

Van der Kolk, Bessel A., Alexander C. McFarlane, and Lars Weisaeth, eds. *Traumatic Stress: The Effects of Overwhelming Experience on Mind, Body, and Society.* New York: Guilford Press, 1996.

Van Dernoot Lipsky, Laura, and Connie Burk. *Trauma Stewardship: An Everyday Guide to Caring for Self while Caring for Others.* San Francisco: Berrett-Koehler, 2009.

Walden, Patricia. "Moving from Darkness into Light." In Cope, *Yoga and Meditation,* 82–97.

Walker, Alice. *The Color Purple.* New York: Harcourt Brace, 1982.

Weintraub, Amy. *Yoga for Depression: A Compassionate Guide to Relieve Suffering through Yoga.* New York: Random House, 2004.

The Welcome: A Healing Journey for War Veterans and Their Families, directed by Kim Shelton. Two Shoes Productions, 2011. Documentary film, www.thewelcomethemovie.com.

White Bison. *The Red Road to Wellbriety: In the Native American Way.* Colorado Springs, CO: White Bison, 2002.

Wilber, Richard. *New and Collected Poems.* New York: Harcourt, 1988.

Williams, Tempest. *When Women Were Birds: Fifty-Four Variations on Voice.* New York: Farrar, Straus and Giroux, 2012.

Yang, Larry, ed. *Making the Invisible Visible: Healing Racism in Our Buddhist Communities,* http://larryyang.org/images/MTIV,_3_ed.pdf.

Zubizarreta, Rosa. "Personal Statement," in Yang, *Making the Invisible Visible,* 31–32.

PERMISSIONS

LIST OF PHOTOGRAPHS

INDEX

ABOUT THE AUTHOR

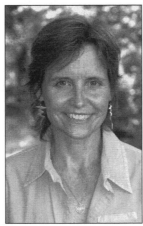

Nancy Vail Shoemaker

Becky Thompson, PhD, RYT-500, is a poet, activist, scholar, and yoga teacher whose work focuses on trauma and healing. She is the author of several books on social justice, including *Mothering without a Compass: White Mother's Love, Black Son's Courage; A Hunger So Wide and So Deep: A Multiracial View of Women's Eating Problems;* and *A Promise and a Way of Life.* Her poetry can be found in her book *Zero Is the Whole I Fall into at Night* as well as in *The Harvard Review, Tidal Basin Review,* and *Sinister Wisdom.*

Thompson is Professor and Chair of the Sociology Department at Simmons College and has taught at Duke University, Wesleyan University, the University of Colorado, Bowdoin College, and elsewhere. In addition to giving lectures and workshops based on *Survivors on the Yoga Mat,* she also teaches yoga at the Dorchester YMCA in Boston and at the Women's International Partnership for Peace and Justice in Thailand. She lives with her marvelous daughter in Jamaica Plain, Massachusetts. Her website is http://beckythompsonyoga.com.

About North Atlantic Books

North Atlantic Books (NAB) is a 501(c)(3) nonprofit publisher committed to a bold exploration of the relationships between mind, body, spirit, culture, and nature. Founded in 1974, NAB aims to nurture a holistic view of the arts, sciences, humanities, and healing. To make a donation or to learn more about our books, authors, events, and newsletter, please visit www.northatlanticbooks.com.